Optom Vision T...

The Need in Minority Populations

James E. Washington, OD, MPA

with Leonard J. Press, OD

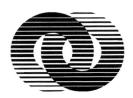

OPTOMETRIC EXTENSION PROGRAM FOUNDATION

Copyright © 2015
All rights reserved. No part of this work covered by the copyright herein may be reproduced or used in any form or by any means—graphic, electronic, or mechanical, including photocopying, recording, taping, or information storage and retrieval systems—without permission of the publisher.

Published by Optometric Extension Program Foundation, Inc.
2300 York Road, Suite 113
Timonium, Maryland 21093
Managing Editor: Kelin Kushin

Library of Congress Cataloging-in-Publication Data
Washington, James E. (James Edward), 1927-2010, author.
Optometric vision therapy : the need in minority populations / James E. Washington ; with Leonard J. Press.
        p. ; cm.
Includes bibliographical references.
ISBN 978-0-929780-44-3 (pbk.)
I. Press, Leonard J., author. II. Optometric Extension Program Foundation, issuing body. III. Title.
[DNLM: 1. Vision Disorders--complications--United States. 2. Health Services Accessibility--United States. 3. Minority Groups--United States. 4. Optometry--United States. 5. Social Problems--United States. WW 140]
RE48
362.197700973--dc23

                        2015018864

****

Optometry is the health care professional specifically licensed by state law to prescribe lenses, optical devices and procedures to improve human vision. Optometry has advanced vision therapy as a unique treatment modality for the development and remediation of the visual process. Effective vision therapy requres extensive understanding of:

- The effects of lenses (including prisms, filters and occluders)
- The variety of responses to the changes produced by lenses
- The various physiological aspects of the visual process
- The pervasive nature of the visual process in human behavior

As a consequence, effective vision therapy requires the supervision, direction and active involvement of the optometrist.

****

Table of Contents

Dedication and Acknowledgements

This book is dedicated to all of those African-American students who did the very best they could but still did not graduate from high school. To all African-Americans who are currently stuck in low-paying jobs because they were not provided with ample opportunities to sustain educational growth. To all of our educators who are doing the best with what they have been given. To those optometrists who practice vision therapy but do not have the support of local school districts and who succeed against improbable odds.

With an undertaking of this magnitude, I must give credit to those who provided the inspiration and courage to proceed in this direction many years ago. Firstly, my teachers: Mrs. Pearl Fisher, Mrs. Halsey, Mrs. Mayo, my English professor at NYU, and the incomparable Countee Cullen—my French teacher who is well-known in the annals of black history.

I also wish to acknowledge my optometric colleagues, Drs. Robert Johnson, Edwin Marshall, Alton Williams, Harold Wiener, and Leonard Press. This is the cadre of folks who have been behind me and with me professionally. A special thank you to my wife, Ethelyn, who is the epitome of the song by the Four Tops when they sing in the vernacular "Ain't No Woman Like the One I Got." As I write this in the 82nd year of my life, I have been blessed many times because I have been surrounded by good friends, and I thank you all for your encouragement.

Special thanks goes to Dr. Edwin Marshall for contributing to the section on Juvenile Delinquency and to my granddaughter Jody Sykes for her help in typing this manuscript. To my grandchildren, Russell III, Partice, and Leslie, and to my great-grandchildren, Jaylin, Nadia, Justin, and Russell IV, I love you all.

About the Author

Dr. James Edward Washington was born in North Carolina and raised in Harlem, New York. He attended DeWitt Clinton High School in the Bronx and Fayetteville University in North Carolina before serving in the United States Army. He received his Doctorate of Optometry (OD) in 1954 from the Northern Illinois College of Optometry and a Master's in Public Administration from Rutgers University in 1983.

A charter member of the National Optometric Association, Dr. Washington served as the second president of the NOA. He was also a member of many other optometric organizations including the American Optometric Association, the College of Optometrists in Vision Development, the New Jersey Society of Optometric Physicians, the Optometric Extension Program Foundation, and the College of Syntonic Optometry.

Dr. Washington practiced optometry in the state of New Jersey for 46 years prior to retiring. He knows first-hand the issues and concerns facing optometrists when dealing with allopathic medicine regarding vision therapy.

Foreword

In 2008, two years prior to his passing in 2010 and just shy of his 83rd birthday, Dr. Washington's wife Ethelyn presented me with the manuscript of a book that Jim had drafted. By this time, Jim's communication skills were seriously impaired, and the draft was accompanied by a note from Ethelyn that read, "Please critique this manuscript for Jim. Any suggestions or ideas will be greatly appreciated." I have done my best and trust that Jim would have been pleased with the result.

The concepts and words you will read in this book stem principally from Dr. Washington, and I am merely here to serve as his voice. I had the privilege of knowing Jim for many years through local, state, and national optometric association meetings. My wife Miriam and I looked toward Jim and Ethelyn as a role model couple in optometry, forging a strong partnership in life outside of our field as well as within the office. We made a point of getting together with them at meetings whenever the opportunity presented itself.

As you will note in these pages, Dr. Washington was passionate about all things related to optometric vision therapy. He considered the effects of nutrition and diet well before it was accepted that these were factors that played a significant role in visual function. He was equally occupied with the visual influences of stress, and though his interests extended to all children, he was particularly concerned about the implications of these lifestyle factors for the African-American community.

Above all, Jim was passionate about education. He was very active in the National Optometric Association and championed the role of vision in education. He was insistent that its members focus not only on eye health issues of particular concern to the African-American community such as glaucoma, but also on visual health issues such as vision-based learning problems. This distinction between eye and visual issues goes well beyond semantics, as you will see within these pages.

In his own quiet way, Dr. Washington was feisty and determined to bring his message to a wide audience. He was part of a long-standing study group of the Optometric Extension Program in New Jersey and was an early adopter of many of the principles he gleaned from the College of Optometrists in Vision Development. He listened intently, and this manuscript represents one of his many ways of giving back. I promised Jim and Ethelyn that in due time I would turn my full attention to bringing his material to publication.

Earlier this year, the President of the National Optometric Association, Dr. Stephanie Johnson-Brown, approached me to be the keynote speaker at the National Optometric Association meeting in 2015, the theme of which is Children's Visual Health. I gladly accepted the invitation as a way, in part, to pay tribute to the influence of Dr. James Edward Washington. The completion of this manuscript is another part of fulfilling my pledge through sharing his friendship, mentoring, and knowledge with the wider audience that he so richly deserves.

One of Dr. Washington's favorite quotes, attributed to George Washington Carver, hinted at Jim's own legacy: *No individual has any right to come into the world and go out of it without leaving behind him distinct and legitimate reasons for having passed through it.*[1]

What you are about to read bears witness to some of the distinct and legitimate principles that guided Dr. Jim Washington on his journey through this world.

Leonard J. Press, OD, FAAO, FCOVD
Fair Lawn, New Jersey
November 2014

on test

Preface

In this twenty-first century, it would seem evident that when the health of our children is at risk, we would be poised to take action. After all, we live in the richest country in the world. A country, I might add, that contains some of the world's brightest minds. Yet somehow we still allow a disproportionate number of our school-aged children to fall through the cracks.

Although many of the topics that we address in this book apply to a wide range of children, I am speaking primarily about African-American students. Our African-American students appear to be on the bottom rung of the education ladder, though this is not uniformly the case. Janice E. Hale, Ph.D. is Founding Director of ISSAC, the Institute for the Study of the African-American Child at Wayne State University's College of Education. Dr. Hale notes that at the outset of school, black students are on par with everyone else, but an achievement gap quickly sets in and progressively rises.

This achievement gap was explored in an article by Fryer and Levitt in *Education Next* (http://educationnext.org/fallingbehind/).

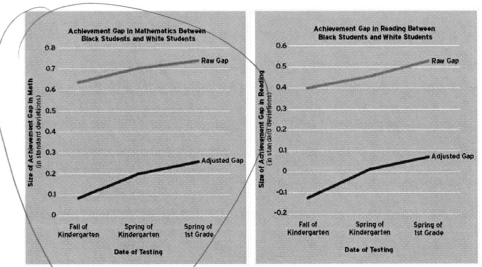

Figure 1: The Raw Gap represents the actual difference in test scores between black students and white students. The Adjusted Gap represents the remaining inter-ethnic test-score gap after adjusting the data for the influence of students' background characteristics.

Black kindergartners and white kindergartners with similar socio-economic backgrounds achieve at similar levels in math and reading. However, both the raw and adjusted gaps grow as students move through school (see Figure 1).

In order to offset this widening gap, Dr. Hale contends that we must do a better job of meeting the needs of diverse learners. In her book *Learning While Black: Creating Educational Excellence for African American Children*, Dr. Hale[2] asserts that the school must become the heart and soul of a broad effort, the coordinator of tutoring and support services provided by churches, service clubs, fraternal organizations, parents, and concerned citizens.

It is my contention that undiagnosed and untreated vision problems represent a significant component of the educational achievement gap in our school systems. While our communities acknowledge the importance of providing minority youth with the type of supplemental help advocated by Dr. Hale, recognition of the role of the visual process has been slow in coming. The first step is to broaden awareness within advocacy circles of the pervasiveness of visually-based learning problems. Now is the time to ratchet up the concerns a notch and pay more attention to visual anomalies that are occurring in near epidemic proportions.

Important as it is, recognition of the problems we face is but one step in a multi-faceted process. We must be more active in developing and bringing effective interventions to our underserved populations. Too many of our children are disengaged from school, and a significant subset of them has visual issues contributing to their disconnectedness. Attention must be paid not only to youths who would otherwise set out on a path to juvenile delinquency, but also in helping talented students realize the full potential of their abilities.

It is time to seal the cracks through which our children fall, and optometric vision therapy is a sealant that is overlooked not only in minority communities, but among the populace at large as well. My aim in writing this book is to share how acute this need is in the populations I served during my 46 years in practice. During that time, the number of children who can benefit from optometric vision therapy has increased for two important reasons:

1) Conditions responsive to vision therapy continually evolve, from developmental delays such as autism, to brain injury (which is on the rise), to sports vision, representing significant opportunities for enhancement.

2) As African-Americans and other minorities within our field avail themselves of this knowledge, the potential supply of suitably-trained professionals able to identify and treat these conditions continues to increase.

Another point to emphasize here is that all too often when I bring up the opportunities available through optometric vision therapy, well-intentioned people dismiss the conversation because they claim that parents or caretakers do not have the time or money to invest in therapeutic endeavors. Certainly there are visual conditions in particular and learning problems in general that will respond best to weekly, office-based interventions. But the umbrella of optometric vision therapy covers territory beyond office- or school-based activities and sessions. Much can be accomplished with the judicious application of lenses and prisms that a child can wear prescriptively. Even when a parent or caretaker has limited resources, third-party coverage is often available for prescriptive lenses, prisms, tints, and sector occlusion.

Any writer struggles at some point with the intended audience for his material. I am not unique in this regard, and my style has focused on prodding you to reflect and then take action on the issues at hand whether you are a parent, an optometrist, an educator, a legislator, or simply—as Dr. Hale would say—a concerned citizen. Please keep the conversation going.

Chapter One

Visual Health

I have long been involved with the National Optometric Association (NOA), a group at the forefront of educating the public about populations who are at higher risk for developing sight-threatening conditions such as glaucoma, diabetic eye disease, and hypertensive retinopathy. We are talking specifically about urban, rural, and minority populations with poor access to eye health care. Efforts oriented toward prevention, early detection, and timely treatment are crucial. Glaucoma is more frequent, more progressive, occurs at an earlier age, and produces more severe consequences in African-Americans than in any other racial or ethnic group. The NOA's "Three Silent Killers" program addresses the importance of prevention and timely care with regard to glaucoma, diabetic eye disease, and high blood pressure—diseases that disproportionately strike minority populations, potentially robbing them of their sight and quality of life.

There is no doubt that these public health initiatives are important, but we may be unwittingly contributing to another problem. In the drive toward preserving sight, we may have lost sight of the fact that eye health is not synonymous with visual health. The eyes can be perfectly healthy and free of disease yet malfunctioning in ways that seriously impair visual development and performance. As we shall see, these distinctions are not a matter of semantics. The eye is a part of the visual system, and a very important part, no doubt. But vision is a process that involves the eyes, brain, central nervous system, and all of the components that make up that system.

One of the more useful definitions of vision, particularly for the purposes of our discussion, was related to me by Dr. Robert "Bob" L. Johnson, a pioneer in optometric vision therapy and the first African-American optometrist to be Board Certified by the College of Optometrists in Vision Development. Bob stated that vision is the process of gathering information into the brain from our various senses, organizing and structuring this information into a conceptual image, and it involves sight, perception, sensory integration, and visualization.

The World Health Organization defines *health*[3] as a state of complete physical, mental, and social well-being and not merely the absence of disease or infirmity. To what extent does vision contribute to this overall state of well-being? It is my contention that sight is linked principally to the physical state of the eye, but vision is a process more intimately related to mental and social well-being. The professional practice of optometry is the examination, diagnosis, and treatment of the visual system. It extends well beyond examination of the eyes to insure eye health and the prescribing of glasses to see clearly, encompassing all aspects of visual health.

From a public health perspective, we have a serious problem in the delivery of professional vision care in the inner cities of our nation. It is a problem that verges on a national crisis, as will be evident in the chapter on juvenile delinquency. The minority health care consumer has limited knowledge as to what constitutes adequate and appropriate vision care. This is compounded by economic pressures and third-party guidelines that abbreviate examination and testing procedures. Access to competent optometric visual care in minority communities is therefore hampered by multidimensional and complex factors, but we may consider them primarily to be:

1. Lack of information available to inner city residents
2. Lack of identification of visual dysfunction amenable to optometric intervention

Patients consult with optometrists as primary eye and vision care providers largely by self-referral. The optometrist recognizes that interdisciplinary care may be required for the patient to receive appropriate services. Components of visual health that optometrists are uniquely positioned to manage include, but are not limited to, the following areas:

- Diagnosis and treatment of refractive and accommodative conditions
- Diagnosis and treatment of problems in eye movements and binocular vision
- Assessment and management of sensory and integrative vision problems
- Evaluation of the patient's interaction with his or her visual environment
- Health counseling and health consumer education

Denis Fisk, Director of Global Clinical Education for Transitions Optical, was on the right track when he authored an article for *20/20 Magazine*[4] on health counseling. Fisk considered healthy sight counseling as a patient-centered approach based on primary care medical methodology. Crucial to the successful implementation of Healthy Sight Counseling is the integration of three key components: Vision Care, Vision Wear, and Education. Healthy Sight Counseling addresses both quantity and quality of vision issues, leading to customized eyeglass prescriptions, where specific eyewear recommendations are made taking into account the individual patient's specific visual needs, occupational and recreational requirements, ocular and systemic health issues, risk factors, and lifestyle.

Fisk's model sets the groundwork for children requiring special considerations in lens prescribing and provides a framework for high-risk patients. Patient awareness and education are viewed as essential components of visual health

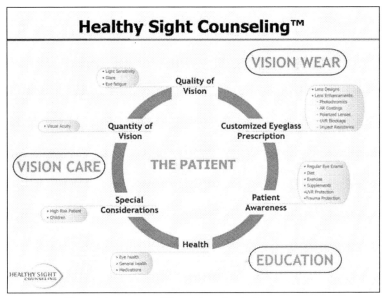

Figure 2: Fisk's model courtesy of Transitions Optical.

maintenance incorporating lifestyle factors such as diet and exercise. While this approach is helpful, it is essentially limited to the physical integrity of the eyes and perpetuates the idea that the key metric of the visual process is Snellen acuity and that the quality of vision is indicated by monocular factors such as contrast sensitivity, night vision, and glare.

A developmental model more relevant to our concerns, and one that builds on the physical integrity of the eyes, was introduced by Dr. Lynn Hellerstein.[5] While acknowledging that physical integrity of the eyes provides a platform for development, Dr. Hellerstein's model emphasizes the importance of visual efficiency, visual information processing, and life activities in overall visual health. She organizes these factors as follows:

Physical Integrity
- Eye health
- Visual pathways
- Eyesight

Visual Efficiency – The 4 Fs
- Fixate
- Follow
- Fuse
- Focus

Visual Information Processing
- Spatial perception
- Eye-hand-body coordination
- Visual memory
- Visualization

Life Activities
- School
- Sports
- Work
- Play
- Relationships

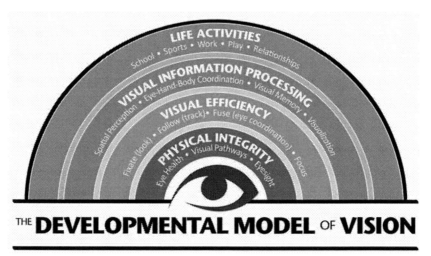

THE DEVELOPMENTAL MODEL OF VISION

Figure 3: Hellerstein's Model

In my experience, this broader view of vision is essential in understanding some of the challenges facing the African-American community. Many of these issues revolve around visual health and are touched upon in a white paper authored by Dr. Joel Zaba reproduced in *Ophthalmology Times*.[6] I want to focus specifically on Dr. Zaba's points relating to school performance and learning, for which he provides ample references. Experts estimate that 80% of what people learn comes through the visual processing of information, yet two-thirds of children in the United States do not receive any preventive vision care before entering elementary school. Once children enter school, the problem only gets worse. Consider the following:

- According to the National Parent Teacher Association, more than 10 million children in this country have vision problems that may contribute to poor academic performance.
- Vision disorders are the fourth most common disability in the United States, and they are one of the most prevalent handicapping conditions in childhood.
- Vision problems are estimated to be prevalent in 25% of all schoolchildren. That is a staggering number of children.
- A study of 5,851 children ages 9 to 15 years indicated that nearly 20% need eyeglasses; yet only 10% of that group had them. Those are pretty sobering numbers.

In school districts in disadvantaged areas, the statistics and research cited by Dr. Zaba are even more alarming.

- In research with Title I students in the fifth through eighth grades and academically and behaviorally at-risk children aged 8 to 18 years, up to 85% of these children had vision problems that were either undetected or untreated.
- Children from poor urban areas, many of whom are members of ethnic minority groups, experience more than twice the normal rate of vision problems. Without the proper vision skills, these children will be at risk of dropping out of high school.
- Teenagers with mediocre high school academic records and low scholastic aptitude test scores have been found to have significant numbers of undetected or untreated vision problems. They are at risk of not completing their college programs.

As you can see, the level of inadequate vision care for children is significant. These unmet needs have consequences that should be of great concern in the African-American community and for society at large. Undetected or untreated visual problems have been linked to high school dropout rates, social and emotional problems, juvenile delinquency, adult literacy problems, and incarcerations. The effect on workforce quality and productivity is evident as well. The time has come for us to seriously address these concerns.

Chapter Two

A Public Health Crisis

In March 2010, Charles E. Basch, Ph.D., a Professor of Health and Education at Teachers College of Columbia University, penned an essay that he dedicated to the urban minority youth of America. Titled *Healthier Students Are Better Learners: A Missing Link in School Reforms to Close the Achievement Gap*, the essay is a Research Initiative of the Campaign for Educational Equity.[7]

Dr. Basch identified seven areas in healthcare as priorities for closing the achievement gap among students. They were selected based, in part, on effectiveness, which is the availability of proven or promising approaches, from a large body of evaluative research. The research had to demonstrate that particular approaches can influence the acquisition and practice of various health-related behaviors. Vision was at the top of his list of priorities as being an educationally relevant health disparity.

It is axiomatic that academic success will be more difficult for a child who cannot see well. However, Dr. Basch emphasizes that even if a child can see clearly, learning-related visual problems can impede learning. He makes the connection that uncorrected hyperopia has been adversely associated with emergent literacy skills, including letter and word recognition, receptive vocabulary, and orthography in children ages 4 to 7 and in lowered reading ability among children ages 7 to 11. Dr. Basch proceeds to review research evidence regarding obstacles to integration between visual sensory perception and the brain that have been associated with educationally relevant outcomes, including binocular coordination of eye movements and stability of binocular control.

Many states require school-based vision screening programs, as do the majority of school districts. More elementary schools than middle or high schools require vision screenings. Among states that require vision screenings, almost all require parental notification of results. Less than half require teacher notification. Teachers are obviously well placed not only to help identify children with learning-related vision problems, but also to encourage children to follow recommended actions (e.g., to wear their glasses as needed). This is, of course, yet another responsibility placed on teachers, which may or may not be reasonable to expect.

There is little data available describing the nature, scope, quality, or yield (i.e., amount of previously unrecognized vision problems that are detected and effectively treated) of school-based vision screening programs. There is no evidence that these programs ensure timely follow-up exams and indicated treatment, an issue known to be especially problematic among low-income families.

I cannot tell you how often parents or caretakers brought children to my office with the misunderstanding that their child had no visual difficulties because they had passed a vision screening administered in the pediatrician's office or by the school nurse. This false sense of security was the centerpiece of a Policy Statement by the American Public Health Association (see Appendix A) advocating that comprehensive examinations are required to adequately address children's visual preparedness for learning rather than reliance upon screening.

Data suggests that low-income children and children experiencing problems in school are disproportionately affected by vision problems. While there are many potential reasons for this, near the top of the list are the increased risks that accompany being born prematurely and at low birth weight, both of which adversely affect eye health and processes associated with the development of vision. Empirical evidence also documents that low-income and minority youth are at greater risk of under-diagnosis and under-treatment of vision problems. This group has a serious need for vision care services which have gone unmet for far too long.

In a nationally representative sample of 48,000+ youth under age 18 cited above from the work of Basch , those from lower income families were less likely to have diagnosed eye conditions than white children and children living in higher income families, perhaps reflecting inequities in access to eye care services. The authors also found that, when diagnosed with eye care problems, black youth living in poverty received fewer and less intensive health care services. These analyses indicate that poor minority youth are both under-diagnosed and under-treated for eye care problems. Local studies support these conclusions. In another national sample of 14,000+ (representing almost 200,000) children with special health care needs, black (8.9%), Hispanic (10.0%) and multi-racial (14.3%) children were two to three times more likely than white children (4.1%) to have unmet vision care needs. The proportion affected by unrecognized or untreated vision problems may also be higher among youth with academic and behavioral risks; sequelae include intellectual disabilities and dyslexia.

Considerable evidence supports the associations between learning-related visual problems and educationally relevant outcomes. Both theoretical and empirical evidence suggests that some of the associations may be causal. Critical visual skills specifically related to learning include tracking (i.e., ability to move across a line of text when reading), teaming or binocularity (i.e., communication between the eyes and the brain), and focusing (i.e., ability to focus accurately at various distances, to change focus quickly, and to maintain focus as long as necessary). Symptoms of visual problems that threaten educational achievement include frequent eye rubbing or blinking, short attention span, avoidance of reading and other close activities, frequent headaches, covering of one eye, tilting the head to one side, holding reading materials close to the face, eyes turning in or out, seeing double, losing place when reading, and difficulty remembering what has been read.

Central to Dr. Basch's research initiatives is the notion of causal pathways, the mechanisms by which health factors influence motivation and the ability to learn. Pertinent to our discussion, there are at least five causal pathways:

1. sensory perceptions
2. cognition
3. school connectedness and engagement
4. absenteeism
5. dropping out

I want to suggest that we pay particular attention to Dr. Basch's notion of connectedness. It is not unreasonable to assume that the child who struggles with vision problems will tend to avoid certain kinds of work because of fatigue, strain, and demoralization. Vision problems cannot be overcome by simply trying harder; they need to be addressed with timely and appropriate treatment. A likely outcome for children demoralized by ongoing struggle coupled with lack of academic success is disengagement from school. A child with an undetected or untreated vision problem is more likely to develop social or emotional problems. Thus, a child's vision problems can affect not only their own learning, but that of their peers. Will address this more in our chapter on vision as related to juvenile delinquency.

Once identified, visual problems need to be corrected. This will not happen without deliberate emphasis on follow-up to receive a comprehensive eye examination and recommended follow-up care. There is an ethical standard that guides against conducting screening programs unless follow-up care is available (American Academy of Pediatrics, 2004), but this appears to be commonly violated with respect to school-based children's vision screening programs. Typically, a positive screening test results in a note being sent home to parents recommending that their child receive an eye examination by an optometrist or ophthalmologist; no further action may be taken. In some contexts, this approach suffices, but this is generally not the case in low-income families.

At least two broad approaches can help increase the chances that referred youth will receive an examination and recommended care. One is intensified outreach to parents to motivate, to enable, and to support them to use existing community-based eye care services. Interpersonal interaction is more likely to be effective than a one-way written communication. Parents should be informed about the nature of their children's vision problem(s), about the potential importance, and about strategies to minimize adverse educational and health effects. Telephone outreach has proven effective in a variety of related applications and warrants consideration here.

Effective programmatic efforts must help ensure that children with these vision impairments receive appropriate treatment in a timely way. For vision problems involving eye-brain or eye-motor system integration, the indicated treatment is often vision therapy. While additional data to support widespread implementation of vision therapy is welcome, there is ample evidence to support its role in improving visual tracking and other visual abilities. Availability and accessibility to such services, and efforts to help ensure high rates of utilization through school-based services or referrals, would be an important innovation. The role of the nurse, other school health service practitioners, or school health program coordinators should be broadened to establish a referral network of vision care services in the community, particularly those serving low-income children.

Chapter Three

Visual Resilience

Chances are you haven't heard of the term "visual resilience" before, and with good reason. To my knowledge, it hasn't been previously written about. But that shouldn't stop us from adopting a term that has significant value in our broader considerations about vision. I'm modeling this after the way in which we use the terms "visual stress" and "visual hygiene."

Visual stress is now a well-accepted term, introduced by Dr. Elliott Forrest, optometrist, to describe factors leading to visual maladaptations. In his brilliant book *Stress and Vision*,[8] published by the Optometric Extension Program Foundation, he relates the more general concepts of stress as introduced by Hans Selye and Walter B. Canon to specific visual conditions induced by these stressors. Visual hygiene is the term used for the set of conditions or modifications used to offset or to lessen the influences of visual stress. Originally associated with Darrell Boyd Harmon, PhD and his work on "The Coordinated Classroom,"[9] the concept has broadened to environmental considerations such as the ergonomics of work stations, postural and viewing angles, optimal lighting, light and color controls of e-Readers, and so forth.

In 2008, the American Psychological Association (APA) released a report from its Task Force on Resilience in Black Children and Adolescents[10] that encourages a shift from an emphasis on risk to exploring the complex interactive process of resilience in African-American youth. The task force offers a vision for optimal development in African American youth within the following five domains:

- Identity Development
- Emotional Development
- Social Development
- Cognitive Development
- Physical Health and Development

For the purposes of our discussion, I'm going to define visual resilience as *resistance to stressors enabling an individual to attain and to maintain optimal visual development.* At first glance, it seems that visual resilience relates most to the Task Force category of Physical Health and Development. Physical development in children and adolescents has received the most attention from the field of Pediatrics and therefore is often considered from the vantage point of disease etiology and treatment. However, as the Task Force report emphasizes, physical development plays an important reciprocal role in other areas of a young person's development, such as those discussed earlier in this report. In other words, we can't treat the five domains above as if they are entirely different areas of development. This fits perfectly within the model of vision espoused by those who practice from the behavioral and developmental optometric models of care.

The brain plays a critical role in the physical development of a child. The endocrine system, which is responsible for the development and release of various hormones that guide physical growth, controls many of the physical changes occurring during childhood and adolescence. The pituitary gland, as part of the endocrine system, controls the secretion of hormones critical to physical growth. The hypothalamus regulates the release of hormones based on a highly sensitized feedback system to control the pituitary. In other words, brain functioning mediates normal physical development in the same way that it mediates all other aspects of development including emotional, social, and cognitive development.

Other examples of mediators of positive physical development covered in the APA Task Force report include good nutrition, physical activity, adequate sleep, and residing in communities devoid of environmental toxins. Enabling resilience requires advocacy at the community and societal levels for access to quality health care and the opportunities for healthy living; specifically in nontoxic environments. The health conditions that disproportionately affect African-American youth include sickle cell anemia, pediatric diabetes, HIV/AIDS, violent injury and death, and obesity. While there is no dispute that these issues warrant the attention that they receive, attention to the effects of undiagnosed or untreated disorders of visual development deserve more serious and widespread attention.

Let me give you an example of an environmental stressor over which we could easily exercise control if we, as a community, chose to do so. The lighting conditions in our school should be part and parcel of proper visual hygiene. This was well-summarized by an engineer from England, Robin Mumford, addressing the influence of lighting on visual stress and performance in an article from Developmental Delay Resources[11] entitled "Lighting and Developmental Delays."

Mumford acknowledges that while the causes of developmental delays are very complex and require intervention on many fronts, simply changing the lighting can be a beneficial addition to other forms of treatment. Many children are excessively sensitive to the quality of the lighting and may overreact.

This hypersensitivity is complicated by visual stress-producing factors that overload their visual environment, confusing their eyes and brains. These factors include the busy and overcrowded conditions that occur in our children's home environments and classrooms. Children are usually unaware of the origin of their discomfort. Environmental stress can contribute to the symptoms of sub-par visual skills that many of these children have such as:

- Rapid fatigue when reading or looking at picture books
- Tendency to lose their place on the page
- Tendency to skim with poor recall of what has been read

- Tendency to read too slowly when processing facts
- Irritated eyes
- Oversensitivity to bright lights

Mumford points out that Dr. John Nash Ott,[12] a pioneer in understanding the relationship between light and health, found that colored filters affect plant growth. He discovered that by using colored filters he could alter a plant's cellular function. He then applied this knowledge to humans. He believes that the light environment in which people live and work affects their biological receptivity. Behavioral problems can thus be a result of poor lighting. The appropriate application of light ranges from influencing Seasonal Affective Disorder to the use of Syntonic Phototherapy to improve visual performance.

Most schools function with fluorescent lights, which lack the balanced spectral aspects of sunlight and increase visual stress factors for many children. Mumford notes that spending an inordinate amount of time under artificial lights may subject children to what another pioneer, Dr. Jacob Liberman, optometrist, calls "malillumination," the corollary of malnutrition. Commonly used fluorescent lights are gradually being superseded by more energy efficient types, some of which claim to be "full spectrum" and more comfortable in use. It is now known that many more factors are involved besides the spectral characteristics making up the color of the light. Features such as glare, simplicity of the lighting, and intensity affect individuals differently. We should embrace any and all factors that may decrease aggressive behavior. Appropriate lighting reduces the visual component of complex stress and provides a calmer environment in which normal function can often become reestablished. Unsuitable lighting can lead to poor reading skill and problematic attention and behavior. This is simply one more of the modern scourges plaguing inner city children.

I want to share with you the example of a resilient child for whom literacy proved to be a path to success. Carolyn Boone, M.D.[13] grew up very poor, but her

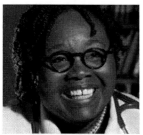

foster mother instilled in her a love of reading. She believed in her, and Carolyn grew up aspiring to achieve great things in part because of all the wonderful role models she accessed through her love of books. As a pediatrician, she now participates in a phenomenal program for her patients called Reach Out and Read, to help pay it forward.

Figure 4: Carolyn Boone, MD

The connection between vision and literacy is so important, yet so many myths and misconceptions about it abound. We are therefore going to devote a good portion of the next chapter to clearing up these misconceptions.

Chapter Four

Visual Performance

For an earlier version of this monograph, my dear friend and colleague Edwin C. Marshall, OD, MS, MPH, former President of the National Optometric Association and champion of diversity throughout Indiana University, contributed a brief overview on vision and juvenile delinquency. Since then, however, he has co-authored a paper of tremendous significance that touches upon juvenile delinquency within a much broader context of visual performance. It dovetails nicely with the concept of visual resilience that we introduced in the previous chapter and speaks to heart of visual literacy.

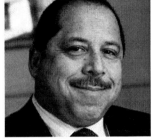

Figure 5: Dr. Edwin C. Marshall

The paper I am referring to is entitled *Through Our Children's Eyes: The Vision Status of Indiana School Children*,[14] co-authored in 2007 by Dr. Marshall with Richard Meetz, O.D., M.S. and L'Erin L. Harmon, M.P.H. It is a report to the Indiana State Health Commissioner and the Indiana Superintendent of Public Instruction. I'll be excerpting a good deal of its introductory material here because it applies to all states, not just Indiana.

Marshall and colleagues note that the lack of preventive eye and vision care for children represents missed opportunities for prevention, early detection, and treatment of health and developmental problems, particularly for children most at risk visually, educationally, and socially. Untreated oculomotor, binocular, accommodative, and perceptual problems interfering with the development of the visual system during early childhood, when the visual system is most susceptible, represent risk factors to serious lifelong visual impairment. These visual problems are potential precursors to poor academic performance, academic drop out, and involvement with the juvenile court system.

The New Jersey Commission on Business Efficiency of the Public Schools[15] issued a report in 2006 concluding that "[c]hildren with reading difficulties who do not receive intervention services are much more likely to be classified as requiring special education than those students with reading difficulties who receive such services," and that children with reading problems fall basically within two groups:

1) Children who have problems mastering basic reading skills and
2) Children with undiagnosed and/or untreated visual problems which prevent them from acquiring reading skills.

The report conservatively estimated that the lack of proper identification and treatment of vision problems cost the state at least $200 million per year in special education services. The argument that we're not doing nearly a good enough job in flagging the unmet visual needs of children languishing in special education is compelling, and it will be well worth your time to read the entire report.

The report by Marshall and colleagues cites two other studies that make compelling points about the visual status of underprivileged children. As reported by Orfield in 2001, an analysis of vision data, standardized test scores, and teacher grades in a low socioeconomic, urban elementary school eye clinic from 1993 to 1999 found that the majority of vision problems were related to near vision and were associated with lower average test scores. The study also found that the interventions of reading glasses and vision therapy correlated with improvements in teacher grades, percentiles, and grade equivalents on standardized tests in reading and mathematics for a school-age population where 85% of the children qualified for free breakfast and lunch.

Now here is a real eye-opening study authored by Wanda Vaughn, OD; W.C. Maples, OD; and Richard Hoenes in 2006.[16] Noting an inverse correlation between visual symptoms and academic performance among third, fifth, and seventh grade public school students, researchers observed that visual factors are better predictors of academic success than race and/or socioeconomic status, even though a majority of academically at-risk students are from low socioeconomic backgrounds. That bears repeating. Visual status is a better predictor of academic success than is race or socioeconomic status.

So there is a double whammy of sorts as summarized by Dr. Marshall and colleagues. The unfortunate dynamic of low socioeconomic status and increased prevalence of undiagnosed and uncorrected vision problems among inner city children helps perpetuate the closed loop of poverty and ill health, exacerbates the negative influence of the social determinants such as education, income, and socialization on the health of children and adults, and burdens the community with societal diseconomies and reduced productivity.

Education rightly occupies much of our attention regarding visual performance in the African-American community. Let's turn our attention to sports for a moment to make a point about helping individuals achieve and perform to their full potential. Larry Fitzgerald is among the elite professional football wide receivers playing the game today, and arguably he is one of the best of all time. Larry's superb visualization and eye-hand coordination is widely acknowledged to be responsible for his considerable athletic talents. Yet as noted by his grandfather, Dr. Robert L. Johnson, Larry first came to him not because of his desire to be an elite athlete, but as an 8-year-old needing optometric vision therapy to help with learning problems. As noted in chapter one, Dr. Robert

Johnson, a dear colleague and second president of the National Optometric Association, was a pioneer in the field of optometric vision therapy. Dr. Johnson recognized that Larry's problems were not because of difficulties with his brain, but in how his eyes communicated with his brain, making it difficult to sustain focus both visually and mentally.

By the time his grandson was 12 and emerging as an athlete, Dr. Johnson tailored many of the vision therapy procedures he was doing with Larry Fitzgerald to athletics. As an example, to improve Larry's precision, control, spatial judgment, and rhythm, Dr. Johnson used an arrangement known as the Marsden Ball Procedure. A ball suspended from the ceiling with painted dots would have to be hit with the corresponding band of color on a rolling pin.

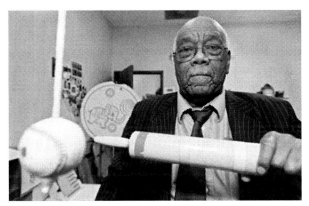

Figure 6: Dr. Robert Johnson

Dr. Stephanie Johnson-Brown, Bob's daughter and Larry's aunt, supervised his vision therapy program. Dr. Johnson-Brown has carried on her father's work in the Plano Child Development Center,[17] focusing on improving visual performance in all facets of life.

The topic of learning related visual problems (LRVPs) folds neatly into the broader area of visual performance. The American Optometric Association has a very useful Quick Reference Guide18 (QRG) to care for this population. The QRG defines learning-related vision problems as deficits in visual efficiency and visual information processing that can interfere with the ability to perform to one's full learning potential. The prevalence of visual efficiency problems in the school-aged population is thought to be in the 15-20 percent range.

The visual deficiencies included in the QRG for LRVPs along with signs and/or symptoms are as follows:

Ocular motility dysfunction

- Moving head excessively when reading
- Skipping lines when reading
- Omitting words and transposing words when reading
- Losing place when reading
- Requiring finger or marker to keep place when reading
- Experiencing confusion during the return sweep phase of reading
- Experiencing illusory text movement; having deficient ball-playing skills

Accommodative-vergence dysfunctions

- Asthenopia when reading or writing
- Headaches associated with near visual tasks
- Blurred vision at distance or near; diplopia
- Decreased attention for near visual tasks
- Close near working distance; overlapping letters/words in reading; burning sensations or tearing of the eyes during near visual tasks

Visual spatial orientation skill deficiency

- Delayed development of gross motor skills
- Decreased coordination, balance, and ball-playing skills
- Confusion of right and left
- Letter reversal errors when writing or reading
- Inconsistent directional attack when reading
- Inconsistent dominant handedness
- Difficulty in tasks requiring crossing of the midline

Visual analysis skill deficiency

- Delayed learning of the alphabet (letter identification)
- Poor automatic recognition of words (sight word vocabulary)
- Difficulty performing basic mathematics operations
- Confusion between similar-looking words (apparent letter transpositions)
- Difficulty spelling non-regular words
- Difficulty with classification of objects on the basis of their visual attributes (e.g., shape, size)
- Decreased automatic recognition of likenesses and differences in visual stimuli

Visual-motor skill deficiency

- Difficulty copying from the chalkboard
- Writing delays, mistakes, confusions
- Letter reversals or transpositions when writing
- Poor spacing and organization of written work
- Misalignment of numbers in columns when doing mathematical problems
- Poorer written spelling than oral spelling
- Poor posture when writing, with or without torticollis
- Exaggerated paper rotation(s) when writing
- Awkward pencil grip

Auditory-visual integration deficiencies

- Difficulty with sound-symbol associations
- Difficulty with spelling
- Slow reading

Visual-verbal integration deficiencies

- Difficulty learning the alphabet (letter identification)
- Difficulty with spelling
- Faulty sight word vocabulary (word recognition)
- Slow reading

Chapter Five

Vision and Acquired Brain Injury

The extent to which even a mild traumatic brain injury (mTBI) can result in visual difficulties has become recognized in optometry since the late 1980s. I bring it up at this juncture because it puts together all of the concepts we've introduced so far in terms of visual health, visual resilience, and visual performance into one clinical entity.

NORA, the Neuro-Optometric Rehabilitation Association, has a wealth of information oriented toward the public.[19] Simply looking at the list of these conditions tells you how many areas of visual function can be impacted by acquired brain injury. Some of the more common issues associated with post-traumatic visual stress are:

- Accommodative Problems
- Binocular Problems
- Eye Movement Disorders
- Problems with Balance and Illusions of Movement
- Reading Problems
- Loss of Visual Field

The Vision Rehabilitation Section of the American Optometric Association recently introduced a Brain Injury Electronic Resource Manual[20] including Visual Dysfunction Diagnosis in Acquired Brain Injury, and the journal *Optometry and Vision Development* has an informative theme issue on the subject.

According to data from the Centers for Disease Control and Prevention,[21] traumatic brain injury poses a significant challenge for African-American communities. African-Americans have the highest death rate from TBI, according to Brainline.org. The TBI rate among African-Americans is higher than for both Hispanics and Caucasians, and one study found that African-Americans were over 2.5 times more likely than Caucasians to be unemployed post-injury according to information cited by Project Empowerment of Virginia Commonwealth University[22] (VCU) in 2011. The information from this Project at VCU is noteworthy because it is funded by the National Institute of Disability and Rehabilitation Research. I am concerned that unaddressed visual sequelae of brain injury contribute to the delayed return toward pre-TBI status.

When brain injury results in visible signs of physical, motor, cognitive, or speech/language impairment, the spotlight of attention is focused on facilitating the patient's recovery. Rehabilitation efforts are typically immediate and intense. What concerns me are the subtle visual signs that often escape detection such as fluctuation in focusing, light sensitivity, problems with movement in crowded spaces, and so forth. These contribute to the delay in being able to return to work for adults or to a normal school load for students. So we're faced with two major challenges, both of which reflect a general lack of knowledge or recognition on the part of the healthcare system, as well as on the part of the patient's caretakers:

1) The under appreciation of visual abnormalities or impairments as lingering signs of acquired brain injury
2) The mistaken belief that visual dysfunctions occurring after brain injury—even visual loss or double vision—will resolve to whatever extent they will with the passage of time and do not warrant active treatment

Nowhere is this lack of awareness greater than in sports, and the implications of this under recognition of mTBI associated with concussions are considerable. This lack of appreciation was recently addressed in Diversity, a publication launched in 1984 as *Black Issues in Higher Education*,[23] focusing on issues pertaining to African-Americans in higher education. When polled, parents of children in higher socioeconomic strata indicate that they are progressively less inclined to allow their children to participate in sports predisposed toward concussions.

Dr. Harry Edwards, a professor emeritus of sociology at the University of California, Berkeley, an expert on African-American athletes and consultant to the San Francisco 49ers and several universities, notes[24] that a large number of college football players are already from minority and disadvantaged backgrounds. If attitudes from current polls hold, there could be fewer whites and considerably more lower-income blacks with limited economic opportunities playing college football. This means that colleges and universities could be dealing with a diminishing number of athletes from which to recruit at the high school level and will dig deeper into the pool for athletes from socioeconomic backgrounds that do not have ready access to the information and process information that would restrict their sons' ability to participate in football. These issues may be compounded by a recent and rather jarring report documenting racial bias in the perception of others' pain that diminishes when objective assessment measures are applied.

To help bridge this gap in awareness, President Obama hosted the Healthy Kids and Safe Sports Concussion Summit in the White House on May 29, 2014. The President noted that concussions can have a serious effect on young, developing brains and can cause short-term as well as long-term problems affecting how a child thinks, acts, learns, and feels. While most kids and teens with a concussion recover quickly and fully, some will have symptoms that last for days, weeks, or months, and a more serious concussion can last longer. You can view the fact sheet based on the Summit here: http://1.usa.gov/1yF6Ytu

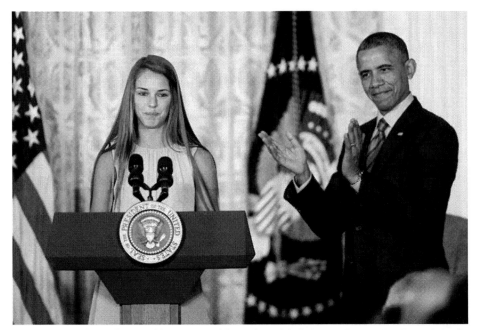

Figure 7: President Obama addressing Healthy Kids and Safe Sports Concussion Summit in the White House, May 29, 2014.

Eye movements have emerged as a particularly sensitive index to cognitive impairment associated with mTBI. The King-Devick Saccadic Test,[25] originally introduced in 1976, has recently emerged in a number of research studies as an adjunct in removal-from-play sideline concussion screening protocols, as well as in aiding clinical decisions about when it is safe to return to play. These tests can be used routinely by athletic trainers as well as by eye care practitioners.

The Centers for Disease Control and Prevention (CDC) has a tremendous array of educational materials online regarding TBI[26] in children tailored to specific groups such as Parents, Clinicians, Youth Sports Coaches, High School Coaches, and School Staff.

As noted in their materials, adults should be alert to the following signs and symptoms:

- Increased problems paying attention/concentrating
- Increased problems remembering/learning new information
- Longer time required to complete tasks
- Increased headache or fatigue during schoolwork
- Greater irritability and/or less tolerance for stressors

Symptomatic students may require accommodations in school, which may be gradually decreased as their functioning improves. Clinicians dealing with children who have visually-related learning disorders will be familiar with these concepts as related to Section 504 Accommodations of the Rehabilitation Act of 1973 for school activities. Until a full recovery is achieved, students may need some or all of the following supports:

- Time off from school
- Shortened day
- Shortened classes
- Rest breaks during the day
- Extended time to complete coursework/assignments and tests
- Reduced homework/classwork load (it is best to specify for teachers the percent of workload that the student can reasonably handle, e.g., 50% homework load)
- No significant classroom or standardized testing at this time

It is important that we make a fuss about these issues, particularly for student athletes who tend to downplay the extent of their mTBI or concussions. Here are some sobering thoughts about the need to break this code of silence and to encourage self-reporting of concussion symptoms. As many as 40% of high school athletes according to a 2013 study,[27] and as many as 78% of university athletes in a 2014 study, may be reluctant to self-report symptoms of a concussion because parents, coaches, or the very culture of the contact or collision sport you are playing encourages you to remain silent in order to:

- avoid jeopardizing your spot in the starting lineup or letting your teammates down;
- avoid being seen as weak or cowardly by your coach and/ or your parents or teammates;
- demonstrate to the coach and your teammates that you can "take a hit like a man;"
- show that you can be as tough as your professional heroes;
- stay in the game and do not want to be pulled out of the game or practice;
- or because you believe that the glory of individual and team success, the promise of a college scholarship, or the lure of a lucrative professional career, is somehow worth the risk of lifetime impairment from continuing to play with concussion symptoms.

In this chapter, I've focused heavily on mTBI in the form of concussions without loss of consciousness because it is so prevalent among our youth. There are many other potential sources of acquired brain injury which should be on our radar. Following developmental timelines, some of the more commonly encountered conditions include:

- Shaken baby syndrome
- Abuse toward children or spouses
- Car accidents
- Strokes or cerebrovascular accidents
- Falls in the elderly

In some instances, there will be objective signs of eye health damage such as change in pupillary responses or hemorrhaging within the eyes or surrounding tissues. In other instances, the signs may be limited to functional performance changes involving visual cognition, or the visual functions listed at the outset of this chapter. The primary role of the clinician with this population, as in all clinical encounters, is to obtain a thorough history, to be conversant with any prior reports, to aid in differential diagnosis, and to be prepared to offer management or treatment strategies as appropriate. Lenses, prisms, filters, and active vision therapy all have a potential role in acquired brain injury. It is merely that the consideration of all these factors is typically more complex in the range of conditions that will be encountered.

Chapter Six

Vision and Developmental Anormalities

The topic of developmental abnormalities covers a very wide area ranging from toxicities such as Fetal Alcohol Syndrome to chromosomal abnormalities such as Fragile X and Down Syndrome to physical challenges of uncertain cause such as Cerebral Palsy. The reader is referred to a wonderful compendium on *Visual Diagnosis and Care of the Patient With Special Needs*[28] that goes into great detail regarding optometric care for special populations.

I want to focus specifically on the subject of Autism Spectrum Disorder (ASD) because it demonstrates some critical principles that I believe cut across many clinical as well as demographic lines. As background reading, the journal *Optometry and Vision Development*[29] has an extensive theme issue on the topic that covers its presumed etiologies, visual symptoms, brain anatomy and electrophysiology of function, insights into diagnosis and treatment, and the role of optometry in early identification.

As reviewed by Gourdine and Algood,[30] information addressing race or ethnicity as related to autism is scant. Research has shown that on average, African-Americans receive a diagnosis of ASD one and a half to two years later than white children. This is significant when we consider the importance of early detection and intervention to long-term outcomes. African-American children are not typically included in research studies that may differentiate phenotypic characteristics necessitating different courses of treatment. Researchers need to be more inclusive of African-American families, listening to their concerns as they describe their child's symptoms, their stresses, and acceptance of the diagnosis of autism.

What might explain the delay in African-American children receiving a diagnosis of autism? Reasons for later diagnosis include a lack of access to quality, affordable, culturally competent health care, according to Martell Teasley,[31] an associate professor in Florida State's College of Social Work. A cultural divide between African-Americans and mainstream health care providers can hinder a timely and correct diagnosis. This is crucial because delayed intervention will result in a poorer developmental outcome that can have a lasting impact on the child's and family's quality of life. The stigma attached to mental health conditions within the black community can contribute to misdiagnoses of autism and underuse of available treatment services.

Toward the end of my career, I acquired a much better appreciation for lifestyle factors and environmental influences. I grew increasingly concerned with their effects on vision in particular and health and disease in general. This has become a hot topic in the field known as epigenetics and gives substance to the holistic approach to development. I'm now going to share with you some information contained primarily in three books that have a holistic bent, the first one related to education and development and the other two related to ASD. The first book is by Antonia Orfield, M.Ed., O.D. titled *Eyes for Learning: Preventing and Curing Vision-Related Learning Problems.*[32] One of my favorite quotes from Dr. Orfield's book is that the best visual systems are made, not born on waves of toxicity. The other two books are by Patricia Lemer, M.Ed., NCC, M.S., one titled *Envisioning a Bright Future* and the second *Outsmarting Autism.*[33]

Autism has been acknowledged as a clinical entity for 70+ years but remains as a multifaceted condition surrounded by confusion and controversy. Such confusion and controversy has spawned an integrated approach between successful activist parents, allied health professionals, physicians, and researchers. They have found that dietary modifications and supplements may hold a partial answer. For example, refined sugars such as glucose and fructose seem to exacerbate problems.

Some foods may cause oxidative stress and inflammatory conditions which we should seek to eliminate or at least to minimize. It is well known that the incidence of preventable chronic diseases is disproportionally high among African-Americans and can be reduced through dietary interventions.[34] Although the role of nutrition in ASD is not as yet certain, there is ample evidence that dietary influences will play a significant role. Gastrointestinal bacterial load appears to be significantly higher in children diagnosed as having ASD, and bolstering digestive enzymes seems to be on the right track toward attacking that problem. Probiotic replacement because of the overuse of antibiotics appears to be a promising approach.

"Total load" is a term used by Patricia Lemer as the aggregate of burdens and challenges contributing to ASD. These include but are not limited to physical and emotional stressors, nutritional deficiencies and excesses, toxic exposures and body burden, and impoverished learning environments. Martha Herbert, Ph.D., M.D., a pediatric neurologist and neuroscientist at the Massachusetts General Hospital and Harvard Medical School, supports Patricia Lemer's concept of total load. In her book *The Autism Revolution,*[35] Dr. Herbert points out that the brain and motor system of children with ASD may create a lot of problems with the use of the eyes as well as other senses, and she notes the contributions of developmental optometry in this regard.[36]

A study by Rhonda Patrick, Ph.D. and Bruce Ames, Ph.D. of Children's Hospital Oakland Research Institute (CHORI) demonstrates the impact that Vitamin D may have on social behavior associated with ASD. Dr. Patrick and Dr. Ames show that serotonin, oxytocin, and vasopressin, three brain hormones that affect social behavior, are all activated by vitamin D. Autism, which is characterized by abnormal social behavior, has previously been linked to low levels of serotonin in the brain and to vitamin D deficiency. This becomes of particular concern when we consider that vitamin D deficiency is considerably more prevalent in the African-American population. According to the U.S. Centers for Disease Control's *Second National Report on Biochemical Indicators of Diet and Nutrition in the U.S. Population*,[37] 31% of African-Americans have a vitamin D deficiency as compared to only 4% of the Caucasian population, with other sources indicating that the prevalence may even be greater.

I have mentioned Patricia Lemer several times, and an organization of which she was the founder, Developmental Delay Resources,[38] is a wonderful source of online information about exogenous and endogenous factors in developmental disorders in general, including vision and autism.

In addition, DDR subsequently partnered with Epidemic Answers,[39] which has carried on the tradition of good information about vision as related to neurodevelopmental disorders in general and ASD is particular.

Chapter Seven

Vision, Juvenile Delinquency, and Literacy

Minority youth are disproportionately represented throughout juvenile justice systems in the United States. African Americans, Hispanics, Asians, Pacific Islanders, and Native Americans comprise a combined one-third of the nation's youth population, yet they account for over two-thirds of the youth in secure juvenile facilities.[40] Various explanations have been put forward for the disproportionate representation of minorities in the juvenile justice system. These range from socioeconomic issues to jurisdictional issues, including police practices to perceived racial bias in the system. Anything that can be done to improve the risk factors for delinquency would be a tremendous service to the individual and the community. I will address these issues again in the concluding chapter on solutions to visual problems. Our first order of business, however, is to establish the linkage between untreated vision problems and juvenile delinquency.

One of the first sources to address vision and juvenile delinquency was an article authored by the developmental optometrist Dr. David Dzik. (Dzik D. Vision and the juvenile delinquent. J Am Optom Assoc 1966;37:462-8.) Over the past 30 years, another optometrist, Dr. Joel Zaba, has been very influential in establishing the connection between visual problems and juvenile delinquency. I therefore want to quote from an excellent review paper he authored for the *Journal of Behavioral Optometry* in 2001:

> *Research in the late 1960s and the 1970s, with the juvenile courts, psychology, and optometry collaborating, indicated a significant number of children with learning disabilities were appearing in the juvenile court system. A relationship was found to exist between juvenile delinquency, learning problems, and associated visual problems. An additional factor now had to be considered: the emotional problems that can be associated with undetected visual problems. As more research was conducted in the 1980s and the 1990s, a much clearer picture was developing, one that showed that a relationship existed between vision, learning disabilities, and juvenile delinquency. By the year 2000, it was accepted that a significant number of undetected visual problems could be found in the population of adjudicated juveniles.*

Regarding vision and illiteracy, Dr. Zaba writes:
> *Research in the early 1990s showed a link between undetected vision problems and illiteracy. This is not to say that every illiterate adult has a vision problem; however, a significant number of them were failing vision screening tests being*

conducted throughout the country. In New York City, 66% of the illiterate adults, in one study, failed one or more parts of an optometric evaluation. In Norfolk and Virginia Beach, Virginia, 74% of an illiterate adult population failed one or more parts of a visual screening program. The illiterate adults failed not only tests measuring distant visual acuity, but they also failed a significant number of tests measuring other visual skills.

The issue of the *Journal of Behavioral Optometry*[41] in 2001 containing Dr. Zaba's paper showcased a landmark conference at the Harvard Graduate School of Education on Visual Problems of Children in Poverty and Their Interference with Learning.

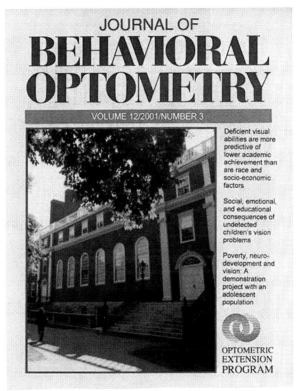

Figure 8: Cover of the issue of the Journal of Behavioral Optometry referred to in the text.

Optometrists' Network has an excellent summary of the Harvard Conference held on April 4, 2001. "It's time we had a discussion between people concerned about vision and people concerned about education," said moderator Gary Orfield, Professor of Education and Social Policy at Harvard University. Antonia Orfield, an optometrist specializing in vision therapy at the Harvard University Health Services Eye Clinic and chief investigator of the Boston Mather School

Inner-City Vision and Learning Project, emphasized the epidemic proportions of visual problems in urban poor children. She noted that 53% of the children tested at the Mather School had visual problems that could affect their ability to read.

Dr. Rochelle Mozlin, Associate Clinical Professor of Optometry at the State University of New York, spoke about her research on vision problems among urban adolescents at risk for dropping out of school and the difficulties in delivering treatment. In two inner city high schools, 52% of the students tested failed the vision screening. Turning diagnosis into treatment proved difficult, because parents and students usually failed to follow up in spite of repeated offers of free services. In the end, only 17 of the 62 students designated as priority cases received the vision care they needed.

Dr. Robert H. Duckman, Professor of Optometry at the State University of New York, summarized his research on vision problems in foster care children in New York City.[42] The results were eye opening:

- Only 16.5% of the 351 children tested had no visual problems at all
- 29.5% of the children had at least three types of visual problems
- 34.6% of the children had vision problems which had previously gone undiagnosed but which probably existed at the time of their last vision screening

Dr. Duckman's conclusion was that the screening now being provided to this population was not sufficient to identify their problems. Rick Weissbourd, a lecturer at Harvard Graduate School of Education, noted that vision problems in learning need to get on policymakers' radar screens. Policymakers concerned with reading simply don't concern themselves much with vision.

Charles Brittingham, President of the Wilmington, Delaware branch of the NAACP, was amazed to discover how vision problems contribute to high school dropout rates, juvenile delinquency, and prison recidivism. He learned about this on a yearly visit to his optometrist Dr. Alton A. Williams, a lifetime member of the NAACP. Realizing that these vision problems can be treated, and how this treatment changed the lives of children academically, behaviorally, and even emotionally by receiving optometric vision therapy, Mr. Brittingham crafted a Resolution regarding the importance of this connection. The resolution acknowledged the role that vision therapy can play in reducing the high rate of recidivism and encouraged members to take aggressive action to have Vision Therapy included in all re-entry programs for formerly incarcerated persons. The resolution passed unanimously at the state level, and Mr. Brittingham then brought the resolution to the national level, raising it at the 100th Anniversary Convention of the NAACP. The NAACP resolution[43] called for its members and units to educate the community, elected officials, and correctional facilities about the merits of optometric vision therapy in helping to reduce the recidivism rate in some prisoners, thereby increasing opportunities for persons reentering society. Once again, the resolution passed unanimously.

We'll conclude this chapter by listing some alarming and sobering statistics, followed by an encouraging study. By no means am I claiming that vision holds the key to profound changes in these numbers. What am I saying is that anything that we can do that has been overlooked is worth trying at this point. Visual dysfunctions and their remediation certainly qualify in that regard. Here are statistics[44] that should give us significant concern:

- 54% of African-Americans graduate from high school, compared to more than three quarters of white and Asian students.
- Nationally, African-American male students in grades K-12 were nearly 2½ times as likely to be suspended from school in 2000 as white students.
- In 2007, nearly 6.2 million young people were high school dropouts. Every student who does not complete high school costs our society an estimated $260,000 in lost earnings, taxes, and productivity.
- On average, African-American twelfth-grade students read at the same level as white eighth-grade students.
- The twelfth-grade reading scores of African-American males were significantly lower than those for men and women across every other racial and ethnic group.
- Only 14% of African-American eighth graders score at or above the proficient level. These results reveal that millions of young people cannot understand or evaluate text, provide relevant details, or support inferences about the written documents they read.
- The majority of the 2.3 million people incarcerated in U.S. prisons and jails are people of color, people with mental health issues and drug addiction, people with low levels of educational attainment, and people with a history of unemployment or underemployment.

Now to end on a comparative high note, with information from a study by optometrists Dr. Wid Bleything and Dr. Sandy Landis involving troubled youth based on results of the COVD-QOL. The College of Optometrists in Vision Development (COVD) developed a multi-domain Quality of Life (QOL) outcomes assessment consisting of 30 questions (COVD-QOL). This establishes the impact of intervention not only on vision, but also on the physical/occupational, psychological, and social effects that are generally associated with impaired visual skills and vision perception difficulties.

The study results[45] that follow were from data collected in a project to examine the feasibility of a vision intervention program within the Oregon Youth ChalleNGe public high school operated by the National Guard near

Bend, Oregon. One of 30 such programs in the United States, these schools were authorized by Congress in 1993 to address the needs of an increasing high school dropout population. The socially at-risk population in this study involved children between 16 and 18 years of age with academic performance between four to six grade levels below expectations.

After being referred to the study, the children received any appropriate lens prescriptions and were then assigned to either a vision therapy or control group. The study was not designed to tease out the relative significance of receiving a lens prescription prior to being assigned to one of the two groups, but specifically to look at whether optometric vision therapy could meaningfully impact the children's quality of life. Vision therapy consisted of two one-hour sessions per week over the course of 12 weeks, with sessions involving the types of procedures that we'll discuss in the next chapter. The control group received extra instruction in the subjects that were being taught in school so that both groups got the same amount of time devoted to their betterment. Results indicated that both groups improved on the COVD-QOL to a statistically significant level, with improvement relatively greater in the group that received optometric vision therapy.

Chapter Eight

Optometric Vision Therapy

In this chapter we'll focus on the need for optometric vision therapy in the African-American Community in terms of its potential to improve visual performance and lessen the sub-optimal experiences of our youth in educational settings, societal functioning, and workplace opportunities. First, let's look at how optometric vision therapy is defined.

The American Optometric Association[46] defines vision therapy and its applications as follows:

Vision therapy is a sequence of neurosensory and neuromuscular activities individually prescribed and monitored by the doctor to develop, rehabilitate, and enhance visual skills and processing. The vision therapy program is based on the results of a comprehensive eye examination or consultation and takes into consideration the results of standardized tests, the needs of the patient, and the patient's signs and symptoms. The use of lenses, prisms, filters, occluders, specialized instruments, and computer programs is an integral part of vision therapy. The length of the therapy program varies depending on the severity of the diagnosed conditions, typically ranging from several months to longer periods of time. Activities paralleling in-office techniques are typically taught to the patient to be practiced at home, thereby reinforcing the developing visual skills.

Research has demonstrated that vision therapy can be an effective treatment option for:

- Ocular motility dysfunctions (eye movement disorders)
- Non-strabismic binocular disorders (inefficient eye teaming)
- Strabismus (misalignment of the eyes)
- Amblyopia (poorly developed vision)
- Accommodative disorders (focusing problems)
- Visual information processing disorders, including visual-motor integration and integration with other sensory modalities
- Visual sequelae of acquired brain injury

Let's use the study by Bleything and Landis with which we ended the previous chapter as the basis for what a typical vision therapy program might encompass. Bear in mind that in that study, as with all vision therapy programs, an appropriate prescription was given to the child first when indicated.

Ocular Motility or Eye Tracking

Example: Hart Chart Saccades, such as identifying first letter and last letter on each row of a letter chart.

O F N P V D T C H E
Y B A K O E Z L R X
E T H W F M B K A P
B X F R T O S M V C
R A D V S X P E T O
M P O E A N C B K F
C R G D B K E P M A
F X P S M A R D L G
T M U A X S O G P B
H O S N C T K U Z L

Figure 9: Hart Chart used by many optometrists for many different types of activities.

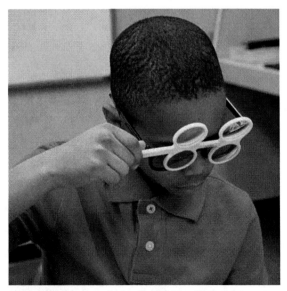

Figure 10: Accommodative Facility or alternately stimulating and relaxing focus

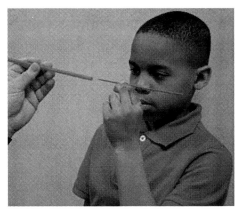
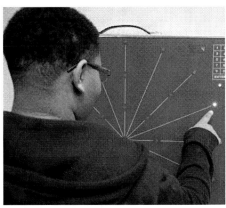

Figure 11: Hand/Eye Coordination or visual guidance of hand movements

Figure 12: Ocular Motility with the saccadic fixator

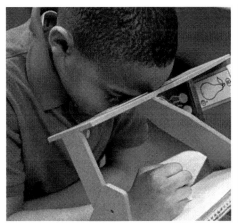
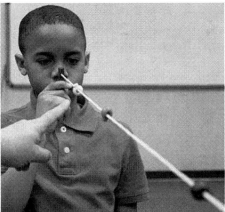

Figure 13: Cheiroscopic Tracing or binocular control of hand/eye coordination

Figure 14: Brock String to work fusion and vergence or eye teaming accuracy and efficiency

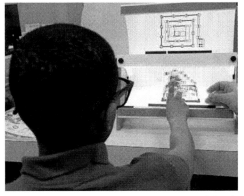

Figure 15: Stereopsis/Vergence or two-eyed depth perception judgment

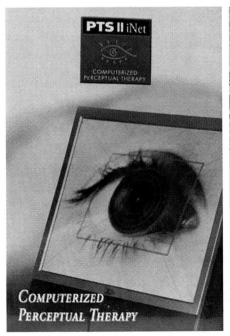
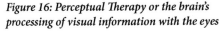
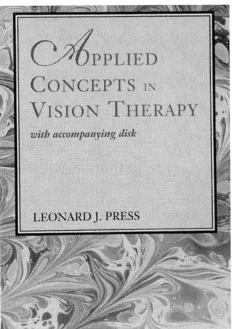

Figure 16: Perceptual Therapy or the brain's processing of visual information with the eyes

Figure 17: Book by Dr. Len Press, "Applied Concepts in Vision Therapy"

There are many resources available now that go into great detail regarding the procedures pictured on the previous page. One of the better sets of references in the public domain are those on Clinical Practice Guidelines published by the American Optometric Association. Here are the links to key Guidelines:

1) Care of the Patient with Accommodative and Vergence Dysfunction[47]
2) Care of the Patient with Strabismus: Esotropia and Exotropia[48]
3) Care of the Patient with Learning Related Vision Problems[49]

There are textbooks available that are entirely devoted to optometric vision therapy such as Applied Concepts in Vision Therapy.[50] These are oriented toward professionals rather than to the public.

The Optometric Extension Program Foundation (OEPF) has considerable information including a compendium of professional papers.[51] I want to highlight one of those papers, *Learning Related Visual Problems in Baltimore City – A Long Term Project*,[52] by Dr. Paul Harris. Aside from the data contained in the project, conducted in the inner city of Baltimore, a self-critique pointed out a number of the challenges in conducting a successful vision therapy program within the school system. We can distill the following principles from the self-critique of the research:

1) Vision therapy as offered through the school system involves compromises. Instead of weekly in-office therapy coupled with assigned daily home therapy, school-based therapy was compressed into a daily school program.

2) New trainees were used in contrast with the type of seasoned therapy environment one typically encounters in private practice.

3) Lack of understanding on the part of the children. This includes what the program was about, why they were chosen to be involved, and what benefits they would derive.

4) It is important to connect the vision therapy with classroom experiences.

5) The vision therapists had no feedback on the optometric and school performance data of the children regarding progress evaluations and transfer.

6) The children tended not to comply with wearing their lens prescriptions. Bear in mind that these stress-relieving lenses often do not result in any immediate sensation of improvement to the child.

7) Because of random assignment to the vision therapy versus control groups, some children in the research group may not have needed vision therapy. The extent to which one benefits from vision therapy involves professional judgment on indications for therapy.

There is a considerable amount of information available through the internet regarding optometric vision therapy that is pertinent to, but extends beyond, the African-American community. These global issues, as covered in White Papers[53] issued by COVD, are as follows:

- School Vision Screenings

- Vision Skills

- Strabismus and Amblyopia

- Myopia (Nearsightedness)

- Reversals

- Vision and Learning

- Vision and Dyslexia

- Bifocals for Children

- What is Optometric Vision Therapy?

- Referral Protocol—Ethics

- Vision Based Learning Problems:
  The Role of the Optometrist on the Multidisciplinary Team

- Vision and Autism

- The Distinction Between Vision Therapy and Orthoptics

Let's backtrack for a moment to point out that optometric vision therapy should never be implemented until the patient has first had a comprehensive eye health and vision examination. In years past, this may have been clouded by issues regarding access and the ability of the family to afford even a basic eye examination. This has now been addressed by the Affordable Care Act, with comprehensive eye examinations for children covered as an essential benefit. Our colleague, Dr. Edwin Marshall, who I cited in Chapter Four, is a member of the National Commission on Vision and Health (NCVH) that issued an important fact sheet on Children's Eye and Vision Care as an Essential Health Benefit.[54] You can access that fact sheet by following the link in the footnote.

Chapter Nine

Hale and Hearty Solutions

It would be sufficiently productive in writing this if all I were to accomplish is to raise awareness in our communities of issues that need to be addressed, but I am looking for us to do more. The time has come to move beyond discussion of the problems and to shed light on their potential solutions. In the Preface to this monograph, I introduced you to the work of Janice E. Hale, Ph.D.; her book *Learning While Black: Creating Educational Excellence for African-American Children* had significant influence on my thinking. Although the book dates back to 2001, many of its issues and suggestions remain quite timely today. Dr. Hale's work is monumental because it breaks the silence on unspoken truths in the African-American community. I am going to put an exclamation mark on some of her observations and suggestions and apply them specifically to the topics addressed in my preceding chapters. At some point in the future, I would like to see Dr. Hale and all educators specifically include visual issues in their discussions.

Too many African-American students remain at the bottom of the education ladder, cannot read adequately, and fail to achieve within the standard curriculum. Parents have a critical role in the education of African-American students. While much of what I have to say relates to remediation, and to African-Americans in poorer socioeconomic environments, we should not lose sight of the opportunities for enrichment so that our children can make full use of their potential. I am also not losing sight of the opportunities for optometric vision therapy to benefit a wider range of patients than emphasized here. Although we are primarily focusing on childhood development and education, there are other areas of concern in our communities such as post-trauma visual stress (alluded to in Chapter Five) and the need for visual rehabilitative therapy in the elderly which we have not touched upon at all.

So what are some of the unspoken truths as related to optometric vision therapy and the need for these services in the African-American community? I will use Dr. Hale's terminology for each of these category headings.

1) **Educational Psychobabble** – This is the term that Dr. Hale uses to describe test results and terms thrown at her by her own child's private school to justify their perception of why he was an underachiever in the early grades. Approximately 65% of African-American families are headed by females, in contrast to 17% of Caucasian-American families, and Dr. Hale was a single mother raising a child who she sent to private school. She does not absolve parents of the obligations to be

more involved in what occurs in the classroom, despite the challenges of balancing work obligations and child rearing responsibilities. Taking matters into her own hands, she rejected the notion that her son would not be a reader or that he had to be medicated for ADHD. Although we do not have any evidence that Dr. Hale's son experienced visual problems, many children fall through the cracks of our educational system because their visual problems remain either undetected or untreated.

2) **In Loco Parentis** – The school exercises their authority over the child by this term which means "in place of the parents." What Dr. Hale suggests is that an In Loco Parents Committee is needed. All too often this arises when a child is failing in public school, and the Child Study Committee or some similarly named group of professionals conducts a psycho-educational evaluation that may lead to an Individualized Education Plan (IEP). In most states, recognition of the role of vision is glaringly lacking. The state of California is relatively unique in that optometric vision therapy is recognized as one of the basic needs that can impact learning, and this should serve as a model for other states to follow.

3) **Waldorf School** – This school model embraces multisensory learning. It combines looking with feeling with action and a lot of hands-on activities. Clearly vision has a large role to play in multisensory learning, as approximately 80% of what we learn is mediated by the visual system. While Dr. Hale does not specifically advocate for Charter Schools, this is an option to which I remain open. While I am not claiming that charter schools are a panacea, they do open the door for teaching strategies that incorporate principles of visual learning such as Integrated Smart Schools.[55]

4) **Culturally Appropriate Pedagogy** – Dr. Hale identifies what she terms African-American teaching strategies. These include: kinesthetic and affective orientation, orality and literacy, vervistic and dynamic activities, and emphasis on the creative arts. Think about the typical learning environment. "Verve" would not be the first word that comes to mind, which Hale identifies as a propensity for relatively high levels of stimulation and for action that is energetic and lively. A significant component of vision is movement, and optometric vision therapy can be a potential bridge to learning based on the fundamentals of "Thinking Goes to School" as outlined by Wachs and Furth.[56]

5) **Intrinsic Motivation** – Hale asserts that African-American children will generally thrive in a setting that uses multimedia and multimodal teaching strategies. They also favor instruction that is variable, energetic, vigorous, and captivating. Look again at Chapter Four and our discussion of the approach that Dr. Bob Johnson took with his grandson, Larry Fitzgerald. The procedures often involved rhythm and movement together with visual spatial judgment and eye-hand coordination. They were directed at visual learning in a way that tapped into the individual's propensity to explore.

There is a wonderful establishment in the vicinity of where I practiced in New Jersey called the Liberty Science Center.[57] While Dr. Hale notes that the average African-American child is raised in a cultural environment that favors creative arts, the Center emphasizes hands-on learning suitable for STEM: Science, Technology, Engineering, and Mathematics. Computer-based technology adapted to optometric vision therapy now makes it possible to transfer visual readiness skills for a wide variety of learning to both the classroom and "real-world" environments. For many African-American children, competitive game-like activities provide a higher degree of intrinsic motivation than what is typically presented in a public school classroom setting.

6) **Cooperative Learning** – Hale observes that African-American children learn best when their learning is oriented toward people rather than objects. They tend to respond best when taught in small groups and with a great deal of nurturing interaction between the teacher and the child and among peers. Experience tells us that this is the antithesis of what goes on in most classrooms. In contrast, during optometric vision therapy, this is often the case. The ratio of therapist to patients is typically in very small groups, if not one-to-one. There is considerable observation and feedback between therapist and patients. One could make the argument that African-American children will actually benefit by having a small group ratio of say two or three patients at a time, above and beyond a one-to-one ratio. Even when there is a one-to-one ratio, learning in a blooming environment with others around but similarly engaged may fuel more effective learning experiences.

7) **Gardner's Multiple Intelligences** – The cultural modalities that we have been considering should, according to Hale, be developed in accordance with Howard Gardner's theories of multiple intelligences.

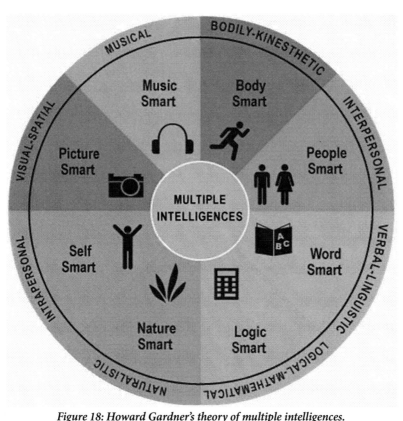

Figure 18: Howard Gardner's theory of multiple intelligences.

Most intelligence tests are heavily weighted toward written linguistic skills and logical-mathematical or computational intelligence. In contrast, Gardner cites strong evidence that human beings have a range of intelligences and that strength or weakness in one intelligence does not predict strength or weakness in any other intelligences. These intelligences can be assessed in common sense ways, or through more formalized test batteries. The eight intelligences are Visual-Spatial, Musical, Bodily-Kinesthetic, Interpersonal, Verbal-Linguistic, Logical-Mathematical, Naturalistic, and Intrapersonal. With regard to optometric vision therapy, the visual-spatial domain holds special significance. Many of the principles used in therapy tap into multiple intelligences, as reflected in the work of Furth and Wachs laid out in *Thinking Goes to School.*[58]

More recently, Wachs has paired with Wieder to author *Visual/Spatial Portals to Thinking, Feeling and Movement: Advancing Competencies and Emotional Development in Children with Learning and Autism Spectrum*

Disorders. This book incorporates a visual-spatial-cognitive manual that is a treasure trove of vision therapy activities compatible with Hale's theories, and consistent with the concept of multiple intelligences.[59]

8) **Counseling and Guidance** – As the saying goes, it takes a village to raise a child. Dr. Hale devotes an entire chapter in her book to the role of the African-American church in creating the village. She cites sources to bolster her tenet that the church is both a preserver of the African-American heritage and an agent for reform. Black churches are a major institutional presence in the black community, serving as a focal point for social salvation as much as religious salvation. One of our colleagues, Dr. Alton Williams, has written a book[60] about the role of God and spirituality in his calling, leading him to provide optometric vision therapy to the benefit of African-American youth in his community.

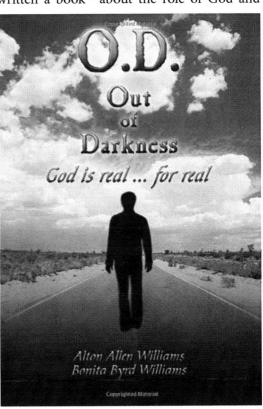

A non-denominational, non-profit agency that offers parenting skills training groups in its counseling programs is COPE. The acronym stands for Counseling, Outreach, Prevention, and Education. I was very impressed with the COPE Center in the vicinity of where I practiced optometry in Essex County, New Jersey. If you don't have a COPE agency in your area, please consider being an agent of change, and offer to help form one. You can contact COPE at: http://www. copecenter.net. In delivering

Figure 19: Dr. Alton Williams' book, "O.D. Out of Darkness"

effective vision therapy services, it is imperative that the child is engaged in the activities, procedures, and guidance provided by the optometric staff. Whether it is through the church, an agency like COPE, or a mentor program, parents can seek out a good role model to help their child benefit from therapy services.

Epilogue

I will close by offering a parallel between societal multicultural diversity and pro-fessional multiculturalism. For a variety of reasons, optometric vision therapy has never been warmly embraced by the eyecare and educational communities. I will go so far as to say that certain medical organizations have practiced a form of bias in discriminating against the evidence accepted for clinical interventions in medicine and the evidence for vision therapy, which is held to a different standard. It is time for allopathic medicine to drop its pretense of self-proclaimed superiority in an aspect of vision development and rehabilitation that optometry has pioneered. Pediatricians and pediatric ophthalmologists cannot and should be not be expected to have expertise in optometric vision therapy. The public will be best served when all of the professions involved in early childhood development, learning, and rehabilitation learn to work together in the patient's best interests.

What needs to be done is for a coalition of professionals with representation from optometry, education, allied therapies, and community enthusiasts to strategize about how we engage the African-American community in awareness about vision therapy. We are in an educational crisis with public health care implications. Too many of our children are not learning, and too many of our young adults are not productive because they lack the tools to succeed. There must be a shared sense of urgency among African-Americans that more people in our communities access vision care, specifically in the form of optometric vision therapy when indicated.

Consider this Success Story:[61]
"Vision Therapy has helped to give Tiffany confidence in herself. Before VT, she had a very hard time reading. What she read, she did not comprehend. It took us three hours every night to do simple school work. Last year in 4th grade, she had all Cs and Ds, which she worked very hard to get. Since VT, she is now getting all A's and B's, and she very seldom brings home any school work at all. Last school year she yelled, screamed, and cried when she had to read. Now she really enjoys reading and is bringing books home all the time. Tiffany's teacher says it's like night and day; the difference in her comprehension has made our lives a whole lot easier. Thanks to Vision Therapy, Tiffany now has confidence and motivation to learn."

I'm not sure what appropriate price tag we can put on optometric vision therapy services. I do know what price we pay, as a community, when children like Tiffany are left to wallow in low self-esteem, struggle with literacy, and fail to become productive members of society.

References

References with internet locations have shortened URLs for your benefit. Often URLs are so long that accurately typing them would be laborious. We've made it easier by giving you shortened addresses, please see below.

1. May 25, 1915 "George Washington Carver – In His Own Words", ISBN-10: 0-8262-0785-5 Page 1

2. http://amzn.to/1yFouhc

3. http://bit.ly/1G6RPsB

4. http://bit.ly/19Lbmkt

5. http://bit.ly/1CUlToJ

6. http://bit.ly/1GOX3YZ

7. http://bit.ly/1F63KBi

8. http://bit.ly/1MFurGH

9. http://bit.ly/1F63LoX

10. http://bit.ly/1CB9dlo

11. http://bit.ly/1I7kBKr

12. http://bit.ly/1GjDhEs

13. http://bit.ly/1y2xd2l

14. http://bit.ly/1F63T80

15. http://bit.ly/1I7ndI2

16. Vaughn, Maples, Hoenes. The association between vision quality of life and academics measured by the College of Optometrists in Vision Development Quality of Life questionnaire. Optometry 2006;77:116-23.

17. http://bit.ly/1yFv1s7

18. http://bit.ly/1DrkLez

19. http://bit.ly/1bQKD7t

20. http://bit.ly/1I7nH0W

21. http://bit.ly/TBIbluebook

22. http://bit.ly/1NDMPKY

23. http://bit.ly/1NKAoPB

24. http://bit.ly/1BR0mZi

25. http://bit.ly/1F67mDt

26. http://1.usa.gov/1NKAy9x

27. http://bit.ly/1CeiHiG

28. http://bit.ly/1xDqpaR

29. http://bit.ly/1NDNs7l

30. http://bit.ly/1IrzTGC

31. http://fla.st/1amQfWl

32. http://bit.ly/1BTwbSh

33. http://bit.ly/1ITXX5C

34. http://1.usa.gov/1NKAOWc

35. Herbert, Martha, "The Autism Revolution: Whole-Body Strategies for Making Life All It Can Be", Ballantine Books, 2012 ISBN-10: 0345527194 ISBN-13: 978-0345527196

36. http://bit.ly/1EKs54Z

37. http://1.usa.gov/1MFyNxw

38. http://bit.ly/1BR1lIS

39. http://bit.ly/1Hmn4gu

40. http://bit.ly/1FlhB9C

41. http://bit.ly/1BTwM6n

42. http://bit.ly/1BR1EDA

43. http://prn.to/19LnRfC

44. http://to.pbs.org/1BTx25n

45. http://bit.ly/1I7p6oc

46. http://bit.ly/1CejYX1

47. http://bit.ly/19LYLx1

48. http://bit.ly/1yFzhrw

49. http://bit.ly/1xDsdke

50. http://bit.ly/1k4VGY6

51. http://bit.ly/1GP2rLI

52. http://bit.ly/1xDsnIf

53. http://bit.ly/1xDst2r

54. http://bit.ly/1NDOv7x

55. http://bit.ly/1NKBn2g

56. http://bit.ly/1EKtQyZ

57. http://lsc.org/for-educators/

58. http://bit.ly/1EKtQyZ

59. http://bit.ly/1MFAzyx

60. http://amzn.to/1CUvsnC

61. http://bit.ly/1NKBw5Q

Appendix A

AMERICAN JOURNAL OF PUBLIC HEALTH MARCH 2002, VOL 92, NO. 3
Improving Early Childhood Eyecare

THE AMERICAN PUBLIC HEALTH ASSOCIATION,
Recognizing that visual development from birth through school age has sensitive and critical periods where abnormalities can lead to permanent impairments, especially in the development of binocular vision, an important part of human vision; and

Realizing that conditions such as strabismus (ocular misalignment) including esotropia (crossed eyes) and exotropia (outward turned eyes) occur in up to 6.7% of children prior to age 5[1-5] and anisometropia (significant difference in refractive prescription between the eyes) has a 1% prevalence[3-6] and clinically significant hyperopia (farsightedness) a prevalence of 3-6%;[6,7] and

Noting that clinically significant hyperopia causes almost half of all cases of esotropia and over 90% of cases of anisometropia, and that these and strabismus are responsible for nearly all amblyopia, the leading visual impairment in children, with a prevalence of up to 4.5%;[2-9] and

Noting that the majority of eye and vision conditions in infancy and preschool ages are not obvious on gross examination and go undetected until children can read standard letter acuity charts around age 5 years;[2,4,5,10] and

Noting that decreased binocular vision and depth perception can lead to problems in gross motor and fine motor development, and that uncorrected hyperopia is associated with deficits in visual perceptual skills, reading readiness, intelligence quotient, and reading achievement,[11-19] and correction of hyperopia by age 4 improves the expected reading achievement later in school;[20] and

Realizing that infant and early comprehensive childhood eyecare is a neglected area, that less than half of pediatricians perform even limited vision screenings,[21] and pediatric screening when performed is usually limited to a light reflex test which will not detect most strabismus, hyperopia, or anisometropia; and

Noting that despite previous APHA resolutions[22,23] and United States Public Health Service Preventive Services Task Force Guidelines,[24] there is a paucity of public health preschool vision screening programs and those programs that exist have low sensitivity and specificity for the above conditions;[25] and

Recognizing that the American Academy of Pediatrics,[26] the American Academy of Ophthalmology,[27] the American Association for Pediatric Ophthalmology and Strabismus,[28] the American Optometric Association,[29] the U.S. Public Health Service,[30] and Prevent Blindness America[31] agree that screening under age 3 is not successful, but there is ample evidence that amblyogenic conditions should be detected and treated as early as possible; and

Realizing that despite intensive efforts to develop eye screening devices such as photorefraction there is at this time no valid screening method for detecting most strabismus, amblyopia, and hyperopia prior to age 5;[4,32,33] and

Noting that reducing blindness and vision impairment in children ages 17 years and under is an objective in Healthy People 2010;[34] therefore

1. Encourages a regular comprehensive eye examination schedule as opposed to just screening based on the onset of strabismus and amblyopia should be set, so that all children have exams performed at approximately age 6 months, 2 years, and 4 years;
2. Encourages all children's health insurance programs to provide vision care benefits;
3. Encourages health insurers to educate parents on the value of adhering to the comprehensive eye exam schedule through the use of health care providers, health education, and health promotion professionals as an important part of preventive health care just as vaccination, physical exam, hearing, and dental exams are;
4. Encourages pediatricians to recommend all children receive exams which have the ability to detect all cases of strabismus, amblyopia, and refractive errors, and refer children at high risk including but not limited to children born prematurely, children with developmental deficits, and children with family histories of strabismus and amblyopia;
5. Requests all children's health programs require monitoring in their quality assurance programs to insure that young children's eye and vision needs are met.

References

1. Stidwill D. Epidemiology of strabismus. Ophthalmic Physiol Opt 1997;17:536-9.

2. Moore BD. The epidemiology of ocular disorders in young children. In: Eye care for infants and young children. Boston: Butterworth-Heinemann, 1996:21-30.

3. Lennerstrand G, Jakobsson P, Kvarnstrom G. Screening for ocular dysfunction in children: approaching a common program. Acta Ophthalmol Scand 1995;77:26-38.

4. Hatch SW. Ophthalmic research and epidemiology. Boston: Butterworth-Heinemann, 1998:193-228,265-8.

5. Blohme J, Tornqvist K. Visual impairment in Swedish children. III. Diagnoses. Acta Ophthalmol Scand 1997;75:681-7.

6. Kleinstein RN. Vision disorders in public health. In: Newcomb RD, Marshall EC, eds. Public health and community optometry, 2nd Ed. Boston: Butterworth-Heinemann, 1990:109-25.

7. Moore B, Lyons SA, Walline J, et al. A clinical review of hyperopia in young children. J Am Optom Assoc 1999;70:215-24.

8. Newman DK, East MM. Prevalence of amblyopia among defaulters of preschool vision screening. Ophthalmic Epidemiol 2000;7:67-71.

9. Dell W. The epidemiology of amblyopia. Problems in Optom 1991;3(2):195-207.

10. Arnaud C, Baille MF, Grandjean H, et al. Visual impairment in children: prevalence, aetiology and care, 1976-85. Paediatr Perinat Epidemiol 1998;12:228-39.

11. Grisham JD, Simons HD. Refractive error and the reading process: A literature analysis. J Am Optom Assoc 1986;57:44-55.

12. Grosvenor T. Refractive status, intelligence test scores, and academic ability. Am J Optom Physiol Opt 1970;47:355-61.

13. Hoffman LG. The relationship of basic visual skills to school readiness at the kindergarten level. J Am Optom Assoc 1974;45:608-13.

14. Williams SM, Sanderson GF, Share DL, Silva PA. Refractive error, IQ, and reading ability: A longitudinal study from age seven to 11. Devel Med Child Neurol 1988;30:735-42.

15. Solan HA, Mozlin R, Rumpf DA. Selected perceptual norms and their relationship to reading in kindergarten and the primary grades. J Am Optom Assoc 1985;56:458-66.

16. Scheiman MM, Rouse MW. Optometric management of learning-related vision problems. St. Louis: Mosby Year-Book, 1994.

17. Rosner J, Gruber J. Differences in the perceptual skills development of young myopes and hyperopes. Am J Optom Physiol Opt 1985;62:501-4.

18. Rosner J, Rosner J. The relationship between moderate hyperopia and academic achievement: how much plus is enough? J Am Optom Assoc 1997;68:648-50.

19. Rosner J, Rosner J. Some observations of the relationship between visual perceptual skills development of young hyperopes and age of first lens correction. Clin Exper Optom 1986;69:166-8.

20. Committee on Practice and Ambulatory Medicine. Vision screening and eye examination in children. Pediatrics 1986;77:918-9.

21. Wasserman RC, Croft CA, Brotherton SE. Preschool vision screenings in pediatric practice: a study from the pediatric research in office settings (PROS) network. Pediatrics 1992;89:834-8.

22. APHA Resolution 8203: Children's Vision Screening. APHA Public Policy Statements, 1948 to present, cumulative. Washington, DC: APHA, current volume.

23. APHA Resolution 8905: Children's Preschool Vision and Hearing Screening and Follow-Up. APHA Public Policy Statements, 1948 to present, cumulative. Washington, DC: APHA, current volume.

24. United States Public Health Service. Vision screening in children. Am Fam Physician 1994;50:587-90.

25. Preschool Vision Screening: Maternal and Child Health Bureau and National Eye Institute Task Force on Vision Screening in the Preschool Child. Pediatrics 2000;106:1105-16.

26. American Academy of Pediatrics Committee on Practice and Ambulatory Medicine, Section on Ophthalmology. Eye examination and vision screening in infants, children, and young adults. Pediatrics 1996; 98:153-7.

27. American Academy of Ophthalmology. Pediatric Eye Evaluations. Preferred Practice Pattern. San Francisco: American Academy of Ophthalmology, 1997.

28. The American Association for Pediatric Ophthalmology and Strabismus. Eye care for the children of America. J Pediatr Ophthalmol Strabismus 1991;28: 64-7.

29. American Optometric Association Consensus Panel on Pediatric Eye and Vision Examination. Optometric clinical practice guidelines: pediatric eye and vision examination. St. Louis: American Optometric Association, 1994.

30. U.S. Public Health Services Task Force. Guide to clinical preventive services, Second Edition. Washington, DC: U.S. Department of Health and Human Services, 1996.

31. Gerali P, Flom MC, Raab EL. Report of Children's Vision Screening Task Force. Schaumburg, IL: National Society to Prevent Blindness, 1990.

32. Cooper CD, Gole GA, Hall JE, et al. Evaluating photoscreeners II: MTI and Fortune videorefractor. Austral N Zealand J Ophthalmol 1999;27:387-98.

33. Mohan KM, Miller JM, Dobson V, et al. Inter-rater and intra-rater reliability in the interpretation of MTI photoscreener photographs of Native American preschool children. Optom Vis Sci 2000;77:473-82.

34. Bowyer NK, Kleinstein RN. Health People 2010—Vision objectives for the nation. Optometry 71:569-78.

Approved by the APHA Governing Council, October 24, 2001.

Appendix B

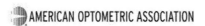

AMERICAN OPTOMETRIC ASSOCIATION

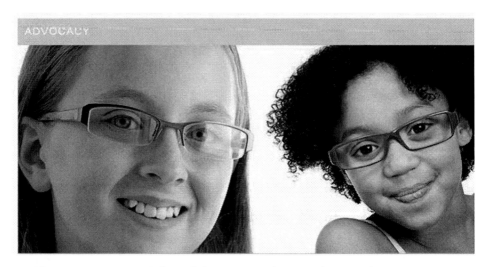

4 Things Parents Should Know About the Pediatric Optometric Care Benefit

As part of the massive health care overhaul, millions of children will benefit from better eye care.

Parents can directly access eye care for their children through their local doctor of optometry.

Optometric eye health and vision care for children has been deemed essential and will be included in new health insurance coverage. This new requirement recognizes that regular comprehensive eye exams during childhood are critical to ensuring visual health and readiness for school.

The AOA is the only national eye health organization Congress and the U.S. Department of Health & Human Services heeded when developing the new requirement. The AOA has been working for years to inform officials and the public about the urgent need for children to have greater access to annual comprehensive eye exams (http://bit.ly/1GgS2JT). Now, the AOA and its members are taking the lead by educating people about how the benefit will work.

Here's what every parent needs to know about the new pediatric optometric care benefit, which will take effect nationwide Jan. 1, 2014:

1. **Your child's coverage is based on a comprehensive eye exam**
   The federal government requires states to define the new benefit as coverage for regular comprehensive eye exams, including all follow-up care and—in almost every case when needed—eyeglasses and contact lenses. This coverage will be included in all health insurance plans sold in health insurance marketplaces (http://bit.ly/1ab5X6u), as well as most new plans sold outside of the marketplaces. Concerned parents covered by health plans delaying a move toward this new standard can contact the AOA Advocacy Group (mailto:MWillette@aoa.org) and urge their employer and plan to make children's eye health care a priority now.

2. **Your child's coverage extends through at least age 18**
   Consistent with the AOA's recommendations, families may use the new coverage for children beginning in infancy and continuing through age 18. A comprehensive eye examination provided by a doctor of optometry, unlike a vision screening, is designed to consistently identify every eye health and vision issue that can affect a child's overall development and achievement.

3. **Your child's coverage is included in your health plan**
   Unlike limited stand-alone plans that can be offered as add-ons to coverage but are not required, the new pediatric eye care essential health benefit will be included as a core benefit and embedded within the overall health plan. This approach provides the seamless primary eye health and vision care children need.

4. **Your child's coverage assures direct access to optometrists**
   Parents can directly access eye care for their children through their local doctor of optometry, both for comprehensive eye exams and needed treatment. When a health plan does not include the family's favorite optometrist in their network, concerned parents can contact the AOA Advocacy Group (mailto:MWillette@aoa.org) and urge insurers to modernize their provider panel by including more optometrists.

Appendix C

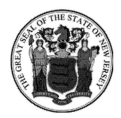

Individual Supportive Education Reform Agenda for New Jersey Reading

Published by the New Jersey Commission on Business Efficiency of the Public Schools on the Topic of Special Education Reform

Spring 2006

Overview of the Commission and its Work

Establishment

The Commission on Business Efficiency in the Public Schools was created in 1979 by the New Jersey Legislature. See P.L.1979, c.69, N.J.S.A. 52:9T-2 et seq. The Commission was given the responsibility to develop and implement a 5-year plan to monitor the implementation of recommendations of the task force on business efficiency and to recommend to the Legislature such statutory changes as may become necessary to facilitate improvements in the business efficiency of the public schools.

Commission Members

The Commission consists of eight members. Currently the members are:

Senator Diane B. Allen
Senator Joseph V. Doria, Jr.
Assemblyman David W. Wolfe
Assemblyman Patrick J. Diegnan, Jr.
Francisco Cuesta
Laurie Fitchett
James H. Murphy
Thomas M. Niland, Ed.D

The Commission Staff

Dennis Smeltzer, Executive Director, (609) 984-1272
http://bit.ly/1HmyFvV

This is the first in a series of reports by the Commission on Business Efficiency of the Public Schools on the topic of Special Education Reform. This report focuses on the impact of the quality of reading education on special education classifications.

SUMMARY

This study included extensive meetings with members of the special education community in New Jersey, individuals involved in this issue in other states, national education research organizations, the examination of legislative activity on this topic in all of the other forty-nine states as well as extensive research of available literature.

One inescapable conclusion of this examination is that children with reading difficulties who do not receive intervention services are much more likely to be classified as requiring special education than those students with reading difficulties who receive such services. The Commission found that if early intervention reading programs with universal screening and follow-up had been available to all of New Jersey's public school children, the State would realize annual cost avoidance in special education funding of $200 Million.

During the course of the examination, the question of the impact that vision care has on reading and thereby on special education classifications was also raised. Studies have indicated that a significant portion of children classified as needing special education had undiagnosed and untreated vision problems, which may affect reading ability. This occurs even though all school age children receive vision screenings as required by law.

As a result the Commission recommends that reading screenings be administered to all first and second grade pupils at the end of the academic year and that remedial reading programs be implemented to correct reading deficiencies. The Commission also recommends that students receive full vision examinations prior to entry to school.

PROBLEM

The focus of the 1997 amendments to the federal Individuals with Disabilities Education Act (IDEA) to ensure the success of students with disabilities and improve their academic achievement is very similar to the goals for which we in New Jersey have struggled. It is important that we accomplish these goals within the effort to provide all students with the highest quality of education possible.

This is important both as a matter of law and because of the strongly held value we in New Jersey place on a quality education for all our children.

It is important to point out that special education programs in New Jersey have accomplished much for students who otherwise would be underserved or not served at all. New Jersey has a long history of progressive thinking and action in the field of special education. The school personnel charged with identifying and providing services to students have a right to take pride in their efforts to provide the best possible education to children requiring special services. Our laws, both as enacted by the Legislature and interpreted by our courts, have always been overzealous in guaranteeing that children needing services receive them. This tradition has produced a culture in New Jersey education that, as a whole, seeks to promote rather than deny special education services.

While this culture is a strength, it has also created rigidity in structure that, at times, prevents flexibility in its operation. One aspect of this problem is the view held by many in the system (teachers, administrators and advocates) as well as clients of the system (students and parents) that the options for assisting a child encountering a reading difficulty are limited. The culture, our funding structure and the range of options available to provide services all contribute to this difficulty.

In the view of the Commission children with reading problems who could avoid later classification through early intervention fall into two groups: (1) children who have problems mastering basic reading skills and (2) children with undiagnosed and/or untreated visual problems which prevent them from acquiring reading skills.

Reading Skills and Special Education Classification. The impact of this changing special education culture on reading seems to have been a decline, over time, of the availability of quality early intervention for students with reading difficulties. Children with reading difficulties have long comprised the single largest portion of students classified as specific learning disabled (SLD). Nationwide some 80 percent of SLD students have primary difficulties with reading. Research indicates that as many as 70 percent of these students would not have been classified had they been appropriately screened prior to first grade and thus received early intervention strategies.[1] Unfortunately under present practice many of these children struggle in traditional classroom programs until they are classified as SLD at the end of second or the beginning of third grade.

Vision and Reading Skills. According to James Kimple.[2]

"Since school tasks rely primarily upon the eyes for acquiring information, it seems logical to make every effort to help (the perceptually impaired) develop their visual skills ... If the child study team refers (the student) for visual examination, the child usually goes to the family physician who just as often returns a report stating that the child has 20/20 vision. The child receives no further help until finally classified... Most of us assume that all children with normal acuity are able to see well enough to do nearpoint work. Nothing could be further from the truth."

He points out that remediation is not likely to improve such a student's academic performance. In this case remediation treats a symptom and not the root problem. It is the visual problem that must be addressed. Considerable research has linked visual skill and reading performance. Many of the correlations are between reading and conditions such as anisopmetropia, binocular coordination, focusing skills, ocular motor efficiency and fixation disparity.[3]

Recent studies looking at learning related visual problems in both "regular" and special needs students has produced interesting results. Studies in Boston,[4] and Baltimore[5] have found that as high as 85 percent of tested children failed at least one screening for a visual problem that could lead to learning difficulty. The highest numbers appear to occur among special education students. Other studies echo these results and show a high occurrence of undiagnosed or untreated visual problems among special education students as well as among the adult illiterate.

In July of 2000 Governor Paul Patton of Kentucky signed into law House Bill No. 706 which requires all to have "a vision examination by an optometrist or ophthalmologist" before entering the public school system. A follow-up study of this legislation was published in the Journal of Behavioral Optometry in 2003.[6] The study examined results on 2,916 children who received vision exams in 2002 including information regarding their history of vision screening during the prior year. This study found that approximately 10.4 of the children had vision problems which went undetected during simple vision screenings but were detected in the more comprehensive vision examination. The study also found that the occurrence of vision disorders in Kentucky matched normal prevalence rates for the children in the general population. Assuming that New Jersey's children also experience disorders in line with the norm, then estimating that 10.4 percent of children entering the public school system also have undiagnosed vision disorders is reasonable. There are roughly 310,000 children enrolled in grades pre-K through third grade (the point at which the second vision screening is due under current law.) Assuming the 10.4 percent estimate above, currently there are 32,000 New Jersey public school students with undiagnosed vision problems, who may not be detected before they reach age 9, attempting to learn to read. After age nine improvements in reading skills becomes extremely less likely for students with reading difficulty. The Commission believes that these children experience a higher likelihood of special education classification than other children.

CURRENT STATUS

Reading Programs. Over the past two years the State has engaged in a more aggressive approach to early literacy. The State has launched the Reading First Program, which has a long range goal of implementing screening and intervention in the early grades in all of New Jersey's public schools. The program includes $10 million per year for four years to fund reading mentors. As of the time of this report Reading First is running in 22 school districts. The New Jersey Department of Education is also making progress in reading programs in the Abbott districts. However, this leaves over 500 school districts without a state supported early intervention reading program.

Vision Programs. Currently the State requires a vision screening of all students as part of required student medical examinations (N.J.A.C. 6A:16-2.2.) This examine is required three times during the child's K-12 schooling: once by the end of third grade, once by the end of sixth grade and once more prior to the end of twelfth grade. The first test focuses on visual acuity but does not test for conditions such as anisopmetropia, binocular coordination, focusing skills, ocular motor efficiency or fixation disparity.

IMPACT OF FAILING TO PROVIDE INTERVENTION ON STATE AID

In New Jersey approximately half of all students with a special education classification are classified as Specific Learning Disabled. That is a little over 100,000 children.[7] Applying the national estimates would indicate 70,000 children with reading difficulties or 56,000 children now classified as requiring special education services who might not be had they received early intervention reading services. This does not include students who could benefit from early intervention reading assistance. There are approximately 200,000 special education students in the State. State aid for special education for the 2003-2004 school year is over $900 million or $4,500 dollars per classified student. (While many affected students will generate other special education funding this analysis uses the tier two amount of $3,329 for calculating savings in table one). Not including local costs, if we had provided these children with appropriate early intervention reading assistance, the savings would be two fold: 1) $200 million dollars per year in special education aid costs, and 2) the rescued lives of thousands of children each year. Per grade level, the savings would be approximately $20 million. Applying this savings estimate to grade levels K-2 would generate $50 million buy the end of the sixth year. Annual savings would then increase each year as these children avoid classification until it reached approximately $200 million per year. The total cost per year for such a program in a state with a similar size population to New Jersey (Virginia) is $22 million including local share. An initial program costing $22 Million could yield cumulative savings of more than one half $Billon within ten years. While New

Jersey has a larger at-risk population, the probable cost of an early intervention program is well under the annual savings.

Table 1. Low end estimate based on tier two funding and no residual savings and no federal funding.

Program year	Annual cost ($Millions)	Annual Savings ($Millions)	Net ($Millions)	Cumulative ($Millions)
Year One	$22	0	($22)	($22)
Year Two	$22	$36	$14	($8)
Year Three	$22	$39	$17	$9
Year Four	$22	$58	$36	$45
Year Five	$22	$80	$58	$103
Year Six	$22	$103	$81	$184
Year Ten	$22	$197	$175	$744
Year Fifteen	$22	$232	$210	$1,773

Table 2. High end estimate based on average aid to capture residual saving and federal funding to cover the cost of the program (in 2001 Dollars).

Program year	Annual cost ($Millions)	Annual Savings ($Millions)	Net ($Millions)	Cumulative ($Millions)
Year One	$0	0	$0	$0
Year Two	$0	$50	$50	$50
Year Three	$0	$53	$53	$103
Year Four	$0	$80	$80	$183
Year Five	$0	$110	$110	$293
Year Six	$0	$142	$142	$435
Year Ten	$0	$272	$272	$1,331
Year Fifteen	$0	$320	$320	$2,903

*The above tables are in 2001 Dollars. Calculations assume a 4 percent growth in SLD placements based on the average change in SDL from 1990-2000 adjusted for tracking changes as well as an aggressive reading campaign in grades 1-3.

Findings

- Approximately half of all New Jersey students with a special education classification are classified as Specific Learning Disabled (SLD).
- The rate of growth in SLD classified children in recent years has been 9 percent while total school enrollment has grown at only 2 percent based on available data.

- Nationwide some 80 percent of SLD students have primary difficulties with reading. As many as 70 percent of these students might not have been classified had they received appropriate early intervention.
- Undiagnosed and untreated vision related learning problems are significant contributors to early reading difficulties and ultimately to special education classification.
- Vision in very young children can change significantly in a one year period.
- The current requirement for vision screening of public school children for acuity only is inadequate.
- The number of students being classified as requiring special education continues to increase.
- Limited alternate intervention options are open to teachers, students and parents to assist a child not thriving under the current approach result in unnecessary classification in special education.
- Over the past two decades programs implemented by reading specialists with young students who demonstrate a difficulty in learning to read have been replaced by full entry into the special education classification system.
- Few students return to full-time general education once classified in special education.
- Current pre-service preparation does not equip teachers to assess reading deficiencies and provide adequate intervention.
- Current staff development does not provide the skills teachers need to assess reading deficiencies and provide adequate intervention.
- The current funding structure does not support intervention remedies to assist reading deficient students short of special education classification.
- The current funding structure draws focus to a limited number of high-cost student placements drawing funds away from early intervention.

Goals for Reform
- Eliminate unnecessary referrals to special education
- Guarantee that any student who can benefit is provided with appropriate support and assistive or remedial services.

Vision
- The Commission on Business Efficiency of the Public Schools has adopted a vision for education of children who encounter learning difficulties: "All of New Jersey's public school students will receive the programmatic support necessary to enable them to achieve at their highest level."

Recommendations

- The State should provide seed money for the implementation of reading screenings and appropriate research-based, early intervention reading programs for pre-Kindergarten through second grade in two pilot districts in each county.
- Require New Jersey school districts to adopt reliable, replicable research based reading programs, one of which must be a systemic phonics based program to be eligible to receive reading program aid.
- Provide reading readiness academies for teachers Pre K-3.
- Refocus pre-service and in-service programs to improve educator's skills in identifying and assisting students with reading difficulties.
- Provide for literacy screening during the Kindergarten year to identify students with reading difficulties.
- The Legislature should require that children present a vision examination certificate signed by an ophthalmologist, optometrist or qualified physician prior to entry into a public school. The report must include the results of a vision examination performed within six months prior the time that a three (3), four (4), five (5), or six (6) year old child is enrolled in a public school, public preschool, or Head Start program. The examination must include measurement of visual acuity in each eye at various distances; assessment of ocular motility and alignment, including eye tracking; strabismus and measurement of actual refractive error; binocular fusion abnormalities; and evaluation of general ocular health, including external assessment.

References

1. Lyon, Fletcher, et al., "Rethinking Learning Disabilities", 2001
2. Kimple, James, "Eye Q and the Efficient Learner", 1997
3. Kulp, M.T, Schmidt, P.P., "Visual Predictors of Reading Performance in Kindergarten and First Grade Children", 1996
4. Orfield, Antonia, OD, MA, FCOVD, "Vision Problems of Children in Poverty in an Urban School Clinic: Their Epidemic Numbers, Impact on Learning, and Approaches to Remediation", 2001
5. Harris, Paul, OD, "Learning-Related Visual Problems in Baltimore City: A Long-Term Program", 2002
6. Zaba, J.N., Mozlin, R, Reynolds, W.T., Insights on the Efficacy of Vision Examinations & Vision Screening For Children First Entering School", Journal of Behavioral Optometry, vol 14/2003/no. 5
7. New Jersey Department of Education, State Special Education Data for 2000-2001

Appendix D

American Academy of Optometry
Binocular Vision, Perception, and Pediatric Optometry Position Paper on
Optometric Care of the Struggling Student
For parents, educators, and other professionals

August 2013

Recent studies have provided new insights into disorders of eye focusing (accommodation) and eye teaming (vergence) that reinforce the need for comprehensive eye examinations and follow-up care for students who are struggling in school.[1-11] These disorders may occur even when individuals have 20/20 eyesight, and can impact students when reading and studying. The typical student with an eye focusing or eye teaming disorder will often experience fatigue, loss of place when reading, and difficulty completing assignments.[1-4] Other common symptoms include skipping small words, rereading sentences, inserting words that do not exist in the text, and experiencing decreasing comprehension the longer that he or she reads.[1,2,5] (See Box 1 for an example). Teachers and parents are often at a loss to explain the source of a student's problems. The difficulties that they observe may not fit exclusively into the currently accepted categories of problems that adversely impact a student's school performance such as a specific learning disability, attention deficit hyperactivity disorder (ADHD), or language-based dyslexia. Parents, teachers and other professionals often have several common questions when seeking information about disorders of eye focusing and eye teaming.

How common are eye focusing and eye teaming problems?

Recent studies suggest that 5-10% of school-aged children have an eye teaming or eye-focusing problem.[6,7,12] Some children report significant symptoms while others experience minimal symptoms. Vision testing that emphasizes a child's ability to read letters on a distance eye chart does not test for eye focusing or eye teaming problems. Even if a child is able to see the 20/20 letters, he or she may have a problem with eye focusing or eye teaming. Additionally, studies have shown that a significant number of students who pass a vision screening for eyesight (ability to see 20/20) have a disorder of eye focusing or eye teaming.[7,12]

When should a student have an eye examination?

The American Optometric Association recommends that school-aged children who have no symptoms have a comprehensive eye examination performed by an eye care professional every two years, while children who have symptoms or are at additional risk for vision problems be examined annually or as recommended.[13] This examination should assess visual acuity (ability to see clearly), refractive status (the need for glasses or contact lenses to see clearly), health of the eyes, as well as eye focusing and eye teaming skills.

Will all eye examinations identify problems with eye focusing or eye teaming skills?

Eye care providers, like other health care professionals, typically use a problem-based approach, yet some may not provide an expanded assessment of eye focusing or eye teaming, especially in cases where the patient does not report specific symptoms. When the parent or student tells the eye doctor that there are difficulties with school performance and requests a comprehensive vision assessment, it is important that the eye doctor perform a thorough evaluation of eye focusing and eye teaming or refer the patient to another doctor who provides this form of care.

What will I observe if my child has eye focusing or eye teaming problems?

Students will often complain of eyestrain, fatigue, blur, words moving, headaches, or loss of place when reading and studying.[1,2,5,7] Parents and teachers may observe behavioral problems affecting school performance such as inattention, avoiding reading and studying, making careless mistakes, and difficulty finishing assignments.[4,8] Visually-related complaints reported by students and their parents are more common in children with eye focusing or eye teaming problems than in those with normal visual skills.[2,4] However the absence of symptoms may be due to avoidance, or lack of awareness on the part of a child as to what it feels like when there is visual stress. Some children who experience symptoms may not complain, because they assume that this is normal.

How are the problems in eye focusing and teaming treated?

Numerous studies have indicated that specific treatment of eye focusing and teaming problems results in a reduction of symptoms and improvement in visual function.[6,9,10,14] In fact, a recent study showed functional neurological changes following treatment with vision therapy for a common eye teaming problem.[15] Treatment can include lenses, prisms, or vision therapy. If a student's problems with eye focusing or eye teaming are found during the eye examination, the intervention program should include a follow-up evaluation to monitor the student's vision status and to ensure that the intervention is successful. Three recent randomized clinical trials have investigated treatments for a common eye teaming problem called convergence insufficiency.[21,22] These studies have shown that office-based treatment with vision therapy is significantly more effective than home-based treatment and that improvement is maintained for at least one year.[9,11,16,23] Some studies have suggested that treatments for eye teaming problems can result in improvements in academic performance such as, reading comprehension, fluency and speed, and attention.[17-20] Parents should discuss treatment options with the eye care provider and understand the advantages and disadvantages of different treatment modalities.

Do all children with vision problems have a learning disability, attention deficit disorder, or dyslexia?

Vision problems can affect students with learning disabilities, language-based dyslexia, or ADHD as well as students without these conditions. Students with learning, reading, or attention problems typically have several factors that impact school performance. Vision problems may be one of these factors and should be treated in these students. Treatment of the vision condition is not intended to cure the learning disability, ADHD, or dyslexia. Instead, the treatment is designed to remove obstacles to efficient learning. For example, if a nearsighted (difficulty seeing far away) student with learning problems had difficulty copying from the board and wearing glasses eliminated this difficulty, it would be clear that the glasses did not "cure" the learning problem; instead, the glasses eliminated a visual obstacle to learning. Similarly, if a student with a reading problem experienced difficulty concentrating on the text due to an eye teaming problem, and concentration improved through glasses, prism, or vision therapy, the treatment did not "cure" the reading disability. Rather, the student was able to sustain concentration comfortably and efficiently thereby benefitting more fully from educational remediation.

SUMMARY

In summary, recent research has clearly shown that problems in eye focusing and eye teaming are common in students and should be evaluated, especially in children who are struggling in school. If a problem is found, then effective treatment should be prescribed. Timely identification and treatment of eye focusing and teaming problems can remove a potential obstacle that may restrict a child from performing at his or her full potential.

An example of a student with an eye teaming problem with 20/20 eyesight who did not need glasses or contact lenses.

Zach is a nine-year old child who was struggling in the first few months of third grade. His teacher noticed him rubbing his eyes during classroom work and he was often the last child to finish his work. He regularly asked to go to the school nurse because of headaches. His teacher also noticed that his oral reading was choppy, although he seemed to be able to decode words and was a good speller.

His teacher asked the school nurse to do a vision screening. The school nurse reported that Zach had 20/20 eyesight in each eye, but she recommended that he have an eye exam because of his headaches. His parents took him to an eye doctor recommended by their pediatrician who reported that Zach's eyes were healthy and that he didn't need glasses. Another health care provider suspected that allergies were the cause of Zach's headaches and suggested allergy testing. As the year progressed, Zach's classroom performance continued to deteriorate. His parents and teacher were concerned about his low reading comprehension score on the mid-year standardized test. Homework was becoming very difficult and Zach became very reluctant to read at home. After his teacher advocated for a second opinion, his parents took Zach to an optometrist who diagnosed him with an eye teaming problem called convergence insufficiency and prescribed optometric vision therapy. Zach received four months of office-based vision therapy supplemented with assigned home therapy, and his parents and teacher noticed significant changes. Of note, he completed his classroom work and homework much faster, no longer rubbed his eyes, read willingly at home and enjoyed it, and his headaches were gone. Nothing had changed in his curriculum or his overall health, but Zach was a more engaged and successful student after the visual problem was resolved.

References

1. Barnhardt C, Cotter SA, Mitchell GL, Scheiman M, Kulp MT, Group CS. Symptoms in children with convergence insufficiency: Before and after treatment. Optom Vis Sci 2012; 89:1512-20.

2. Borsting E, Rouse M, Mitchell G, et al. Validity and reliability of the revised convergence insufficiency symptom survey in children ages 9-18 years. Optom Vis Sci 2003;80:832-8.

3. Chase C, Tosha C, Borsting E, Ridder W. Visual discomfort and objective measures of static accommodation in college students. Optom Vis Sci 2009;86:883-89.

4. Rouse M, Borsting E, Mitchell GL, et al. Academic behaviors in children with convergence insufficiency with and without parent-reported ADHD. Opt Vis Sci 2009;86:1169-77.

5. Sterner B, Gellerstedt M, Sjostrom A. Accommodation and the relationship to subjective symptoms with near work for young school children. Ophthalmic Physiol Opt 2006;26:148-55.

6. Abdi S, Rydberg A. Asthenopia in schoolchildren, Orthoptic and ophthalmological findings and treatment. Doc Ophthalmol 2005;111:65-72.

7. Borsting E, Rouse MW, Deland PN, et al. Association of symptoms and convergence and accommodative insufficiency in school-age children. Optometry 2003;74:25-34.

8. Borsting E, Rouse M, Chu R. Measuring ADHD behaviors in children with symptomatic accommodative dysfunction or convergence insufficiency: A preliminary study. Optometry 2005;76:588-92.

9. Convergence Insufficiency Treatment Trial (CITT) Study Group. Randomized clinical trial of treatments for symptomatic convergence insufficiency in children. Arch Ophthalmol 2008;126:1336-49.

10. Scheiman M, Cotter S, Kulp MT, et al. Treatment of accommodative dysfunction in children: Results from a randomized clinical trial. Optom Vis Sci 2011;88:1343-52.

11. Scheiman M, Mitchell L, Cotter S, et al. A randomized clinical trial of treatments for convergence insufficiency in children. Arch Ophthalmol 2005;123:14-24.

12. Rouse M, Borsting E, Hyman L, et al. Frequency of convergence insufficiency among fifth and sixth graders. Optom Vis Sci 1999;76:643-9.

13. The American Optometric Association Consensus Panel on Pediatric Eye and Vision Examination. Pediatric Eye and Vision Examination. 2nd ed. St Louis, MO: American Optometric Association; 2002.

14. Sterner B, Abrahamsson M, Sjostrom A. The effects of accommodative facility training on a group of children with impaired relative accommodation--a comparison between dioptric treatment and sham treatment. Ophthalmic Physiol Opt 2001;21:470-6.

15. Alvarez TL, Vicci VR, Alkan Y, et al. Vision therapy in adults with convergence insufficiency: clinical and functional magnetic resonance imaging measures. Optom Vis Sci 2010;87:E985-1002.

16. Scheiman M, Mitchell GL, Cotter S, et al. A randomized clinical trial of vision therapy/orthoptics versus pencil pushups for the treatment of convergence insufficiency in young adults. Optom Vis Sci 2005;82:583-95.

17. Atzmon D, Nemet P, Ishay A, Karni E. A randomized prospective masked and matched comparative study of orthoptic treatment versus conventional reading tutoring treatment for reading disabilities in 62 children. Bin Vis Eye Muscle Surg Q 1993;8:91-106.

18. Dusek WA, Pierscionek BK, McClelland JF. An evaluation of clinical treatment of convergence insufficiency for children with reading difficulties. BMC Ophthalmol 2011;11:21.

19. Stavis M, Murray M, Jenkins P, Wood R, Brenham B, Jass J. Objective improvement from base-in prisms for reading discomfort associated with mini- convergence insufficiency type exophoria in school children. Binocul Vis Strabismus Q 2002;17:135-42.

20. Borsting E, Mitchell GL, Kulp MT, et al. Improvement in academic behaviors after successful treatment of convergence insufficiency. Optom Vis Sci 2012;89:12-8.

21. Scheiman M, Gwiazda J, T L. Non-surgical interventions for convergence insufficiency. Cochrane Database of Systematic Reviews 2011, Issue 3. Art. No.: CD006768. DOI: 10.1002/14651858.CD006768.pub2.

22. Lavrich JB. Convergence insufficiency and its current treatment. Curr Opin Ophthalmol 2010;21:356-60.

23. Convergence Insufficiency Treatment Trial Study Group. Long-term effectiveness of treatments for symptomatic convergence insufficiency in children. Optom Vis Sci 2009;86:1096-103.

Appendix E

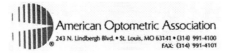

American Optometric Association
243 N. Lindbergh Blvd. • St. Louis, MO 63141 • (314) 991-4100
FAX: (314) 991-4101

Vision Therapy
Information for Health Care and Other Allied Professionals

A Joint Organizational Policy Statement of the American Academy of Optometry and the American Optometric Association

INTRODUCTION

Society places a premium on efficient vision. Schools and most occupations require increasing amounts of printed and computer information to be handled accurately and in shorter periods of time. Vision is also a major factor in sports, crafts, and other pastimes. The efficiency of our visual system influences how we collect and process information. Repetitive demands on the visual system tend to create problems in susceptible individuals. Inefficient vision may cause an individual to slow down, be less accurate, experience excessive fatigue, or make errors. When these types of signs and symptoms appear, the individual's conscious attention to the visual process is required. This, in turn, may interfere with speed, accuracy, and comprehension of visual tasks. Many of these visual dysfunctions are effectively treated with vision therapy.

PERTINENT ISSUES

Vision is a product of our inherited potentials, our past experiences, and current information. Efficient visual functioning enables us to understand the world around us better and to guide our actions accurately and quickly. Age is not a deterrent to the achievement of successful vision therapy outcomes.

Vision is the dominant sense and is composed of three areas of function:

- Visual pathway integrity including eye health, visual acuity, and refractive status.
- Visual skills including accommodation (eye focusing), binocular vision (eye teaming), and eye movements (eye tracking).
- Visual information processing including identification, discrimination, spatial awareness, and integration with other senses.

Learning to read and reading for information require efficient visual abilities. The eyes must team precisely, focus clearly, and track quickly and accurately across the page. These processes must be coordinated with the perceptual and memory aspects of vision, which in turn must combine with linguistic processing for comprehension. To provide reliable information, this must occur with precise timing. Inefficient or poorly developed vision requires individuals to divide their attention between the task and the involved visual abilities. Some individuals have symptoms such as headaches, fatigue, eyestrain, errors, loss of place, and difficulty sustaining attention. Others may have an absence of symptoms due to the avoidance of visually demanding tasks.

VISION THERAPY

The human visual system is complex. The problems that can develop in our visual system require a variety of treatment options. Many visual conditions can be treated effectively with spectacles or contact lenses alone; however, some are most effectively treated with vision therapy.

Vision therapy is a sequence of activities individually prescribed and monitored by the doctor to develop efficient visual skills and processing. It is prescribed after a comprehensive eye examination has been performed and has indicated that vision therapy is an appropriate treatment option. The vision therapy program is based on the results of standardized tests, the needs of the patient, and the patient's signs and symptoms. The use of lenses, prisms, filters, occluders, specialized instruments, and computer programs is an integral part of vision therapy. Vision therapy is administered in the office under the guidance of the doctor. It requires a number of office visits and depending on the severity of the diagnosed conditions, the length of the program typically ranges from several weeks to several months. Activities paralleling in- office techniques are typically taught to the patient to be practiced at home to reinforce the developing visual skills.

Research has demonstrated vision therapy can be an effective treatment option for:

- Ocular motility dysfunctions (eye movement disorders)
- Non-strabismic binocular disorders (inefficient eye teaming)
- Strabismus (misalignment of the eyes)
- Amblyopia (poorly developed vision)
- Accommodative disorders (focusing problems)
- Visual information processing disorders, including visual-motor integration and integration with other sensory modalities

SUMMARY

Vision therapy is prescribed to treat diagnosed conditions of the visual system. Effective therapy requires visual skills to be developed until they are integrated with other systems and become automatic, enabling individuals to achieve their full potential. The goals of a prescribed vision therapy treatment regimen are to achieve desired visual outcomes, alleviate the signs and symptoms, meet the patient's needs, and improve the patient's quality of life.

This Policy Statement was formulated by a working group representing the American Academy of Optometry, American Optometric Association, the College of Optometrists in Vision Development, and the Optometric Extension Program Foundation. The following individuals are acknowledged for their contributions:

Gary J. Williams, OD; Chair

Susan A. Cotter, OD   Louis G. Hoffman, OD, MS   Glen T. Steele, OD

Kelly A. Frantz, OD Stephen C. Miller, OD Jeffrey L. Weaver, OD, MS

Approved by: American Academy of Optometry, May 14, 1999 American Optometric Association, June 22, 1999

College of Optometrists in Vision Development, June 25, 1999 Optometric Extension Program Foundation, June 25, 1999

BIBLIOGRAPHY

American Optometric Association. Position statement on vision therapy. J Am Optom Assoc 1985;56:782-3.

Caloroso EE, Rouse MW, Cotter SA. Clinical management of strabismus. Boston: Butterworth-Heinemann, 1993.

Ciuffreda KJ, Levi DM, Selenow A. Amblyopia: basic and clinical aspects. Boston: Butterworth- Heinemann, 1991.

Coffey B, Wick B, Cotter S, et al. Treatment options in intermittent exotropia: a critical appraisal. Optom Vis Sci 1992;69:386-404.

Cooper J, Medow N. Intermittent exotropia: basic and divergence excess type. Binoc Vis Eye Muscle Surg Q 1993;8:185-216.

Cooper J, Selenow A, Ciuffreda KJ, et al. Reduction of asthenopia in patients with convergence insufficiency after fusional vergence training. Am J Optom Physiol Opt 1983;60:982-9.

Daum KM. The course and effect of visual training on the vergence system. Am J Optom Physiol Opt 1982;59:223-7.

Flax N, Duckman RH. Orthoptic treatment of strabismus. J Am Optom Assoc 1978;49:1353-61. Garzia RP. Efficacy of vision therapy in amblyopia: a literature review. Am J Optom Physiol Opt 1987;64:393-404.

Griffin JR. Efficacy of vision therapy for nonstrabismic vergence anomalies. Am J Optom Physiol Opt 1987;64:411-4.

Grisham JD, Bowman MC, Owyang LA, Chan CL. Vergence orthoptics: validity and persistence of the training effect. Optom Vis Sci 1991;68:441-51.

Liu JS, Lee M, Jang J, et al. Objective assessment of accommodation orthoptics. I. Dynamic insufficiency. Am J Optom Physiol Opt 197956:285-94.

The 1986/87 Future of Visual Development/Performance Task Force. The efficacy of optometric vision therapy. J Am Optom Assoc 1988,59.95-105.

Optometric clinical practice guideline: care of the patient with accommodative and vergence dysfunction. St. Louis: American Optometric Association, 1998.

Press LJ. Applied concepts in vision therapy. St. Louis: Mosby, 1997.

Rouse MW. Management of binocular anomalies: efficacy of vision therapy in the treatment of accommodative deficiencies. Am J Optom Physiol Opt 1987;64:415-20.

Scheiman M, Wick B. Clinical management of binocular vision: heterophoric, accommodative, and eye movement disorders. Philadelphia: Lippincott, 1994.

Suchoff IB, Petito GT. The efficacy of visual therapy: accommodative disorders and non- strabismic anomalies of binocular vision. J Am Optom Assoc 1986;57:119-25.

Wick BW. Accommodative esotropia: efficacy of therapy. J Am Optom Assoc 1987;58:562-6. Wick B, Wingard M, Cotter S, Scheiman M. Anisometropic amblyopia: is the patient ever too old to treat? Optom Vis Sci 1992;69:866-78.

Appendix F

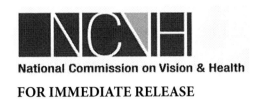

National Commission on Vision & Health

FOR IMMEDIATE RELEASE

Media Contact: Lena Parsons Phone: 312-255-3073
Lena.parsons@hillandknowlton.com

New Evidence-Based Research Shows that Universal Comprehensive Eye Exams Would Help More Children Succeed in School

Only three states require exams, many children remain untreated, creating a new public health concern, according to report from National Commission on Vision and Health

Washington, DC, August 12, 2009 – Even though universal comprehensive eye exams for children prior to starting school would result in more children being diagnosed and successfully treated for vision problems and eye diseases, requirements vary widely from state to state and only three states require eye examinations for school-age children, according to a new report from the National Commission on Vision and Health.

The report, "Building a Comprehensive Child Vision Care System," found that children are being screened at low rates and those who are screened do not often receive the necessary follow-up and treatment they may require. Children without health insurance and those living in poverty are at the greatest risk. Although the majority of states do require some type of vision screening prior to children entering public schools, they often fail to use the best screening tests and to assure important follow-up for those who fail the screening. Only three states, Kentucky, Illinois and Missouri, require comprehensive eye exams for children entering school. Currently fifteen states do not require any form of screenings or exams, resulting in a public health emergency for millions of children.

"Children from low-income families lack the health care resources necessary to break the cycle of poverty," said David Rosenstein, DMS, MPH, Oregon Health & Science University professor emeritus. "This lack of vision care is handicapping our most vulnerable populations. Research from the Centers for Disease Control and Prevention shows that 83 percent of families earning less than 200 percent of the federal poverty level have children who have not seen an eye care provider during the prior year. This must change now for the sake of our children."

According to doctors, early detection and treatment are essential in treating eye diseases and disorders in children and can lead to better school achievement and overall health outcomes which can lead to prevention of eye disease and developmental delays. Vision screenings vary in scope and are not designed to detect many visual problems. A comprehensive exam by an eye doctor does, and an eye doctor can also provide follow-up treatment.

"This report finds that vision screenings are not the most effective way to determine vision problems", said Deborah Klein Walker, EdD., principal author of the report and past-president of the American Public Health Association. "Screenings missed finding vision conditions in one-third of children with a vision problem and most of the children who are screened and fail the screening don't receive the follow-up care they need. This despite the fact that many of the vision problems affecting children can be managed or even eliminated if they receive proper care right away."

Millions of children are without adequate care and preventable eye diseases and correctable vision problems are neglected. Many eye and vision disorders lack obvious signs and symptoms and can be prevented or treated through early detection, follow-up care and ongoing treatment. Undiagnosed and untreated vision problems in children can potentially limit the range of experiences and kinds of information to which the child is exposed. Visual learning plays an important role in how a child learns to understand and function in the world.

Studies indicate that one in four children have an undetected vision problem. Additionally, a quarter of school- age children suffer from vision problems that could have been addressed or eliminated if appropriate eye assessment programs and follow-up care had been in place when they started school.

"Starting school with good vision should be a part of every child's back-to-school plan," said Commission chair Edwin C. Marshall, O.D., M.P.H., Vice President for Diversity, Equity, & Multicultural Affairs at Indiana University. "Clear and comfortable vision is essential for learning, and the country would be well-served to make sure children's eye exams are accessible and required."

Given the data surrounding this public health emergency, the Commission recommends agencies at the federal, state and local levels collaborate with academia, business, providers and the public to create a comprehensive child vision care system to ensure all children are assessed for potential eye and vision problems before entering school and throughout the school years. In addition to universal access to vision care, the Commission recommends a point of accountability within local public health agencies, a national education campaign, and ongoing data collection to monitor the use and efficacy of child vision exams.

Specifically, the commission supports a national child vision care system that:

- Includes child vision health care in key legislation at the federal and state levels.
- Assures adequate comprehensive coverage of child vision care services by all pulic and private insurers and payers.
- Establishes a child vision health categorical program linked to the Title V MCH Block Grant within the Maternal and Child Health Bureau in the Health Resources Service Administration (HRSA), Health and Human Services (HHS).
- Develops a national set of children's vision guidelines for screening and examinations and assure these guidelines are adopted by all states.
- Implements and fund a national clearinghouse for child vision health within the Department of Health and Human Services.
- Enhances and fully funds national campaigns to encourage early identification of child vision problems and to prevent injuries from sports and toys.
- Designs and implements an ongoing data system that monitors prevalence of child vision problems together with access and utilization of child vision care services.
- Develops and facilitates a broad coalition of child-oriented stakeholder groups to work towards the establishment and maintenance of a comprehensive child vision system across the country.

About the National Commission on Vision and Health:
The National Commission on Vision and Health strives to improve the nation's visual health by collaborating with science and health policy experts to ensure informed analysis and policy recommendations in order to prevent blindness improve vision and eliminate vision health disparities. The multidisciplinary commission publishes consensuses reports from its ten-person leadership team, comprised of optometrists, ophthalmologists, a dentist, a physician assistant, a state health department chronic disease program specialist, a Medicaid policy specialist, the executive director of the National Medical Association, and a CDC disabilities specialist. For more information visit www.visionandhealth.org.

Appendix G

Poverty Neurodevelopment & Vision
A Demonstration Project With An
Adolescent Population

Rochelle Mozlin, OD

Originally published in the *Journal of Behavioral Optometry* 2001;12(3).

Abstract

The biosocial consequences of poverty, such as malnutrition, low birth weight, teenage pregnancy and maternal complications of pregnancy, can be related to central nervous system maturation and therefore, to visual development and school achievement. Continuing risks for additional damage to the central nervous system accrue as these children are raised in an impoverished environment. A vision screening of 625 adolescent inner city students demonstrates the vision and learning outcomes associated with poverty. Fifty two percent of the students failed the screening. Of 23 students with hyperopia greater than 2 diopters, 18 or 78 % were special education students. Various intervention strategies were developed to address diagnosed visual dysfunctions, but compliance in this population was very poor. A partnership of optometry, education and public health will be required to develop new programs to identify students with vision problems and provide them with the services they require.

Keywords: adolescent, compliance, hyperopia, neuro-development, poverty, public health, special education, vision screening

Introduction

The impact of poverty on the health and development of children is readily acknowledged. However, the extent of accompanying functional visual and visual-perceptual disorders has not received adequate attention. Although well designed optometric research involving this population of children is lacking, there is extensive research on the impact of biosocial consequences of poverty on neurodevelopment. In particular, malnutrition, low birth weight, teenage pregnancy and maternal complications of pregnancy can all be related to central nervous system maturation and therefore, to visual development and school achievement. These children are born of poverty into poverty. In this hostile environment, we must not overlook the continuing risks for additional damage to the central nervous system,[1] decreased stimulation to developing sensory systems and reduced access to medical care. The results of an expanded vision screening of an adolescent inner city population demonstrates the impact of vision and learning outcomes associated with poverty. It further provides an example of inadequate compliance to address diagnosed visual dysfunctions, and indicates a vital role for optometry, as a member of the school health care team, to render appropriate treatment to economically impoverished and socially disadvantaged children.

BIOSOCIAL FACTORS
Malnutrition

The neonate is expected to survive in the same hostile environment that the mother endured during pregnancy. If we consider adequate nutrition as the engine that drives the child's mental and physical development, then we can appreciate the vicious cycle as a generation of poorly nourished individuals rear their children under conditions predictably destined to produce future generations of malnourished and poorly functioning individuals.[2] Maternal malnutrition increases the risk of a neonate with a low birth weight (LBW), and continued malnutrition reduces the child's resistance to infection.[3] Undernourished hungry children are less alert and offer a diminished response to their environment.[4] Among children ages 2 to 5 years, 13% of those from families below the poverty line were below the 5th percentile in height compared to just 5% of those above the poverty line.[5] When neurointegrative tests were administered, poor children who were short performed below average. Stature was not a factor among children with normal nutrition.[6]

Optometrists are more likely to treat children with subclinical malnutrition, which manifests less severe neurointegrative disorders, but sufficient to produce an impact on classroom performance. Providing 3rd and 4th grade children with breakfast in school resulted in significant improvements in verbal fluency among a population of undernourished children.[7] In addition, malnutrition usually does not occur alone, but in conjunction with low income, substandard housing, familial disorganization, and a climate of social apathy.[8]

Low Birth Weight

The combined effects of low income, inadequate education, and the absence of early prenatal care lay the foundation for adverse birth outcomes among mothers of low socio-economic status (SES). When income is less than 1.5 times the poverty level, the prevalence of LBW is 24% higher than with incomes three times the poverty level.[5] Mothers without high school diplomas have 67% more LBW children than those who attend college.[5] Inner city mothers are 3.3 times more likely to smoke and 3.7 times more likely to use alcohol, when compared to a control group.[9] Cigarette smoking and alcohol consumption have been associated withLBW, prematurity, reading and arithmetic problems, and lower APGAR scores.[10,11]

LBW children who survive have a high prevalence of visual perceptual and cognitive defects. IQ scores decline with decreasing birthweight as do visual-motor integration skills.[12,13] Other visual problems with increased prevalence include strabismus and amblyopia[14] and severe reductions in sight associated with retinopathy of prematurity.[15]

Teenage Pregnancy

The problems accruing from LBW babies are abetted by the persistence of teenage pregnancies. Teenage mothers represent an increased risk of having LBW babies, premature babies and, when compared to 25-29 year old mothers, 68% more babies who die during the first year of life.[16] Thirty-nine percent of teenage girls who are from families who live below the poverty line have a child, compared to 10.4% of those with family incomes at three or more times the poverty line. Poor adolescents are more likely to become pregnant and when they do, they are more likely to have the baby and remain unmarried[17] The consequences of teenage pregnancies have the potential to manifest the same array of developmental and visual problems that result from low birthweight and malnutrition. These children must face an unfavorable environment from which the survivors are unlikely to emerge unscathed.

Maternal Complications of Pregnancy

Maternal complications of pregnancy such as toxemia, hypertension, and bleeding during pregnancy yield a continuum of reproductive casualties which range from fetal and neonatal death and cerebral palsy, at one extreme, to learning disabilities at the other. Towbin stressed that hypoxia is the most common cause of cerebral damage and the degree of damage is related to the extent of the hypoxia.[18] Therefore, the emergent patterns of clinical disability and aberrant academic performance may be more subtle. However, near term, the cortical sites most at risk are those that govern cognition, sensory and fine-motor activity.

The marked effects of SES on complications of pregnancy were reported by Pasamanick, et al.[19] The incidence of bleeding and toxemia increased from 5% to 10% to 22% as one moved from white upper economic fifth to white lower economic fifth to the non-white group. Kawi and Pasaminick[20] compared the hospital records of 205 boys with certified reading disabilities with a matched group of normal readers. In this sample, 16% of the mothers of the disabled readers had two or more complications of pregnancy compared to only 1.5% of the normal readers.

Impact on Visual Development

From the evidence that has been provided, it is reasonable to conclude that malnutrition and undernutrition, low birth weight and prematurity, teenage childbearing, and maternal complications of pregnancy can influence neurointegrative development and functioning. In his review of pre- and peri-natal factors on intelligence, Vernon[21] recommends that specific events should not be viewed in isolation because these variables seem to operate in a multifactorial fashion and interact with both genetic predisposition and environmental factors. Damage to the CNS continues to accrue via mechanisms associated with an impoverished environment, such as a higher incidence of illness, lead poisoning, incomplete immunizations[22] and inequalities in access to appropriate health care services.[23]

The developmental aspects of intersensory and sensory-motor integration in the primary grades have been well documented.[24] Birch and Belmont[25] focused on auditory-visual integration as a neurointegrative task that involves both simultaneous and successive processing and is dependent upon the integrity of the CNS. The ability to treat auditory and visual information as equivalent representations significantly correlates with reading in grades 1 to 6 and is also related to nutritional risk.[26] When combined with the measurement of accurate eye movements (a sensory-motor activity), Solan[27] was able to account for 35% of the variance in reading performance in a population of reading disabled 4th to 6th graders. Kramer's study[28] strongly supports the association between visual-perceptual and academic functioning in children with sociodemographic, family, and health characteristics. Lower scores on cognitive tests such as the Weschler Intelligence Scale for Children-Revised (WISC-R) Block Design and Reading and Arithmetic subtests of the Wide Range Achievement Test (WRAT) were associated with minority status, lower income, and lower educational level of the parent. General health status, history of birth complications and prenatal exposure to smoke were also predictors, but to a lesser extent. In a recent study, Kattouf and Steele[29] found that lower-income public school children scored significantly lower on subtests of the Test of Visual Perceptual Skills (TVPS) than children in private school.

The impact of neurointegrative disorders may not be evident until the child fails to respond to educational challenges in the classroom. Often, the teacher suggests an eye exam, and evidence of these defects are revealed during the visual analysis. Strabismus, numerous less severe binocular anomalies, accommodative disorders and other visually related developmental delays may result from insult to the integrity of the central nervous system.[30]

Vision Screening of an Adolescent Inner City Population

A vision screening project undertaken at an inner city high school in New York City serves to illustrate the visual sequelae of poverty's continuing assault on the our nation's youth.[31] From 1985-87, a vision screening program was performed on 625 high school students as part of a drop-out prevention program. In addition to providing information about students' visual status to parents and teachers, the program was also aimed at educating the teachersabout the role of vision in classroom learning and developing effective intervention and compliance strategies.

Subjects

The 625 students attended inner city high schools in underserved communities in the Bronx and Manhattan. As a service project aimed at drop-out prevention, priority was given to students classified as learning disabled. Hence, 285 (58 %) of the students were enrolled in special education programs. The remaining students were referred either by a teacher, parent or self, on the basis of suspected visual problems or poor academic performance.

Methods

The screening procedures used were based on existing clinical procedures (the Orinda study)[32] and then modified to reflect the greater visual demands, especially near visual activities, inherent in the high school curriculum. The final pass-fail criteria were therefore, more stringent than those that would be applied in the typical elementary school screening program.[33]

Two manpower days per week were devoted to this program from October through May over three school years (1985-88). One of the doctors utilized the time for screening, and consultation with students, teachers and parents, while the second doctor utilized the time for screening, consultation, program administration and development of lectures and workshops.

Results

A total of 327 or 52.3%of the students failed the vision screening. A higher percentage of the special education group failed (56.6 %) than the non-special education group (48.7 %), but the difference was not statistically significant. The greatest number of failures were in the refractive category. Forty-four percent of all the students participating in the screening potentially required glasses, either for distance viewing, reading or both. Of major concern was the large number of uncorrected hyperopic students, who are at great risk for symptoms associated with reading, such as blurred vision, headaches, inability to sustain at reading, and poor comprehension. When "priority cases" of hyperopes (those with uncorrected refractive errors exceeding 2 diopters) were separately considered,

18 of 23 (78 %) of these high hyperopes were special education students. Indeed this difference was statistically significant ($p < .01$).

During the first year of the screening, 126 letters were sent home informing parents of their children's failure and requesting a complete vision examination. Two letters were returned with information from the examining practitioner. During the next school year, more aggressive intervention strategies were developed and targeted at the students classified as priority cases. A paraprofessional and two family workers contacted parents and made appointments for them to speak with the optometrists. Of 37 students classified as priority, 14 appointments were made, seven of these appointments were kept and all seven students received comprehensive vision examinations. During the final year of the screening, priority students were offered appointments at the State University of New York, State College of Optometry's University Optometric Center. Of 13 students for whom appointments were made, 10 received care. Seven received glasses through Medicaid and two were given fee reductions based on financial need. After three years of modifying strategies and focusing our intervention resources on the most needy cases, only 17 of 62 (27 %) of the students received the vision care they required.

Discussion

Traditional models of vision screening programs focus on casting a wide net, identifying children with potential vision problems, and notifying parents of the need for further care. When considering this adolescent population, the conceptual model was changed to reflect a need to concentrate on students at high risk of dropping out because of academic failure. Therefore, we (Suchoff and Mozlin) focused on those students either classified as learning disabled or identified as high risk. As we provided teachers with opportunities to learn about and discuss the visual prerequisites for classroom learning, we defined the mechanism to identify the high risk students. The number of referrals to the vision screening program increased as the teacher education component of the program was accomplished. Our success at identifying students with potential vision problems was confirmed by the high failure rate.

Our model of vision care delivery was far less successful at providing the follow-up care these students required. Our interactions with other professionals indicated that our experience in terms of compliance was not unique. Rather, this represents a public health issue that still has not been sufficiently recognized. In the long run, how this problem is conceptualized will determine the direction and success of remedial efforts.[34] Simply improving access to appropriate healthcare services will not eliminate visual deficiencies in the poor and underserved communities.

The appropriate investment will require new partnerships to develop programs that provide health, social and educational programs that stress the importance of compliance. Successful programs such as Head Start must be expanded to provide services to older children. Appropriate infrastructures and systems will be required to ensure coordination and continuation of services. Innovations and strategies, such as school-based programs,[35] must make these services available to the children, rather than waiting for parents to seek care for their children. A partnership of optometry, public health, and education might well have an impact on the high school drop-out rate by identifying students with vision problems, and providing them with the services they require.[31]

In 1954, the United States Supreme Court, in the landmark case Brown v. Board of Education of Topeka, struck down the concept of "separate but equal." Chief Justice Warren wrote," In these days, it is doubtful that any child may reasonably be expected to succeed in life if he is denied the opportunity of an education. Such an opportunity, where the state has undertaken to provide it, must be made available to all on equal terms ... Separate educational facilities are inherently unequal."[36] Forty-seven years ago, the Supreme Court justices understood the need to invest in the future of all American children. Although our nation's school systems are no longer physically segregated, inequalities still exist which have been created by poverty's continuous assault on neurological integrity and development and the barriers it creates to academic achievement.

This paper was presented at the April 4, 2001, conference, "Visual Problems of Children in Poverty and Their Interference with Learning" held at the Harvard Graduate School of Education.

References

1. Birch HG, Gussow JD. Disadvantaged children: health, nutrition and school failure. New York: Harcourt, Bruce & World, 1970.

2. Winick M. Malnutrition and brain development. J Pediatr 1969; 74:667-679.

3. Pollitt E. Developmental impact of nutrition on pregnancy, infancy, and childhood: public health issues in the United States. In: Bray N, ed. International Review of Research in Mental Retardation, vol 15. New York: Academic Press, 1988:33-80.

4. Connors CK, Blouin AG. Nutritional effects on the behavior of children. J Psychiatr Res 1982; 3 (17):193-201.

5. Klerman LV. Alive and well? A research policy and review of health programs for poor young children. New York: National Center for Children in Poverty, 1991.

6. Birch HG. Malnutrition, learning and intelligence. Am J Public Health 1972;.62:773-84.

7. Chandler AMK,Walker SP, Connolly K, Grantham-MacGregor SM. School breakfast improves verbal fluency in undernourished Jamaican children. J Nutr 1995; 125: 894-900.

8. Wilson A. Longitudinal analysis of diet, physical growth, verbal development and school performance. In: Balderston J, Wilson A, Friere M, Simonen M, eds. Malnourished children of the rural poor: The web of food, health, education, fertility and agricultural production. Boston: Auburn House Publishing, 1981: 39-81.

9. Binsacca DB, Ellis J, Martin DG, Petitti DB. Factors associated with low birthweight in an inner-city population: the role of financial problems. Am J Public Health 1987; 77: 87-102.

10. Johnston C. Cigarette smoking and the outcome of human pregnancy: a status report on the consequences. Clin Toxicol 1981; 18: 189-209.

11. Streissguth AP, Barr HM, Sampson PD. Moderate prenatal alcohol exposure: effect on child IQ and learning problems at age 7 1/2 years. Alcohol Clin Exp Res 1990; 14: 662-9.

12. Wiener G. Rider RV, Oppel WC, Fischer LK, Harper PA. Correlates of low birth weight: Psychological status at six to seven years of age. Pediatrics 1965; 45:433-45.

13. Wiener G. Rider RV, Oppel WC, Harper PA. Correlates of low birth weight: Psychological status at eight to ten years of age. Pediatr Res 1968; 2:110-8.

14. Drillien CM. Prematurity in Edinburgh. Arch Disabled Child 1956; 31:390-4.

15. Dobson V, Quinn GE, Summers CG, Saunders RA, Phelps DL, Tung B, Palmer EA. Effects of acute phase retinopathy of prematurity on grating acuity development in very low birthweight infant. The Cryotherapy for Prematurity Cooperative Group. Invest Ophthal Vis Sci 1994; 35: 4236-44.

16. United States Birth Cohort of 1991. U.S. Department of Health and Human Services, Center for Disease Control and Prevention, National Center for Health Statistics. Linkage Research Group. Personal communication.

17. Facts in brief (Report). New York: The Guttmacher Institute, 1994.

18. Towbin A. Neuropathological aspects: II. Prenatal brain damage and its sequels. In: Black P, ed. Brain dysfunction in children: etiology, diagnosis and management. New York: Raven Press, 1981: 47-77.

19. Pasaminick B, Knobloch H, Lillienfeld AM. Socio-economic status and some precursors of neuropsychiatric disorders. Am J Orthopsychiatry 1956; 26: 594.

20. Kawi AA, Pasaminick B. Association of factors of pregnancy with reading disorders in childhood. JAMA 1958; 166: 1420-3.

21. Vernon PE. The effects of perinatal and other constitutional factors on intelligence. Educ Rev 1979; 31:141-7.

22. Starfield B, Budetti PB. Child health and risk factors. Health Serv Res 1985; 19:817-86.

23. St. Peter RF, Newacheck PW, Halfon N. Access to health care for poor children: separate and unequal? JAMA 1992; 267:2760-4.

24. Solan HA, Mozlin R. The correlations of perceptual-motor maturation to readiness and reading in kindergarten and the primary grades. J Am Optom Assoc, 1986; 57:28-35.

25. Birch HG, Belmont L. Auditory-visual integration in normal and retarded readers. Am J Orthopsychiatry 1964; 34:852-61.

26. Cravioto J, DeLicardi ER. Intersensory development of school-aged children. In: Scrimshaw NS, Gordon JE, eds. Malnutrition, Learning and Behavior. Cambridge, MA: MIT Press, 1968: 252-69.

27. Solan HA, Ficarra AP. A study of perceptual and verbal skills of disabled readers in grades 4,5, and 6. J Am Optom Assoc 1990; 61:628-34.

28. Kramer RA, Allen L, Gergen PJ. Health and social characteristics and children's cognitive functioning: results from a national cohort. Am J Public Health 1995; 85: 312-8.

29. Kattouf VM, Steele GE. Visual perceptual skills in low income and rural children. J Optom Vis Devel 2000; 31:71-5.

30. Hoffman LG. The effects of accommodative deficiencies on the developmental level of perceptual skills. Am J Optom Physiol Opt 1982; 59: 254-62.

31. Suchoff IB, Mozlin R. Vision screening of an adolescent inner city population: a high failure rate and low compliance on follow up care. J Amer Optom Assoc 1991; 62: 598-603.

32. Blum H, Peters H, Betman J. Vision screening for elementary schools: the Orinda study. Berkeley: University of California Press, 1959.

33. Sheedy J, Saladin J. Validity of diagnostic criteria and case analysis in binocular vision disorders. In: Schor C, Cuiffreda K, eds. Vergence Eye Movements: Basic and Clinical Aspects. Boston: Butterworths, 1983.

34. Solan HA, Mozlin R. Children in poverty: Impact on health, visual development and school failure. J Optom Vis Devel 1997; 28:7-25.

35. Krumholtz I. Results from a pediatric vision screening and its ability to predict academic performance. Optometry 2000; 71:426-30.

36. Brown v. Board of Education of Topeka, 347 U.S. 483 (1954).

Corresponding author:
Rochelle Mozlin, OD, FAAO, FCOVD
State University of New York
State College of Optometry
33 West 42nd Street
New York, NY 10036-3610
Date accepted for publication: May 4, 2001

Appendix H

Learning-Related Visual Problems in Baltimore City: A Long-Term Program

Paul Harris, OD

Originally published in the
Journal of Optometric Development 2002; 33(summer).

Abstract

A longitudinal, single-masked, random sample study of children at a Baltimore City Public Elementary school documents the prevalence of learning-related visual problems in the inner city of Baltimore and tests the effectiveness of vision therapy. Vision therapy was provided to one of the randomly selected groups and data was collected on optometric tests, visual performance tests, and standardized achievement tests before and after treatment was provided. Data presented shows that the vision therapy program has made a significant difference in the demand level of reading that could be read for understanding, in math achievement on standardized testing, and in reading scores on standardized testing, as well as on infrared eye-movement Visagraph recordings, which show significant changes on nearly all mechanical aspects of the reading process. This paper makes a strong case that untreated learning-related vision problems are a significant public health concern and that the profession of optometry has a treatment modality that can address these problems in a significant way. The paper presents many of the difficult questions that had to be addressed during both the early formation stage of the study and during the execution of the study. The rationale behind the key decisions that had to be made during each step of the program is provided so that future researchers may be able to replicate this study with full knowledge of what to expect.

Keywords: Learning-related vision problems, vision development, vision therapy, visual training, perception, performance, school-based vision therapy, Visagraph, inner-city, ocular motor dysfunction, binocular dysfunction, visual attention problems, convergence insufficiency.

In 1997 representatives of the Abell Foundation of Baltimore came across an article in the Boston Globe chronicling the work of Dr. Antonia Orfield with inner-city students in Boston. The article started the foundation on a search for information, which led them to investigating to what extent a problem similar to that which Dr. Orfield was addressing in Boston existed in the city of Baltimore. After suitably convincing themselves that a public health problem did potentially exist in the youth of the city of Baltimore, representatives of the Abell Foundation asked me to be the chief investigator for a program that would first identify the prevalence of learning related vision problems in the Baltimore City Public Schools and then test the efficacy of treatment for those conditions identified. At the time I was living in Denmark on a one-year sabbatical to teach behavioral vision care in Europe. The following paper chronicles step by step how I worked toward achieving these goals. The paper describes how the formal research protocols were established, reports the initial data collected on the children, the preliminary data following the first year of the study, and the data at the end of the second year of the study, and then comments on each of the findings in detail.

Many decisions were made at critical steps in the development of the protocols. It is my intent to share the factors that were weighed in each of these decisions so that (1) the reader may fully understand the rationale that went into the choices that were made in the development of the protocol and (2) those who wish may use the information presented here to guide them in making the key decisions necessary to establish similar programs in other communities.

Statement of the Problem

Baltimore, Maryland, "The City That Reads," has had trouble living up to its motto. Like most large cities its public schools have lagged behind in basic academic achievement as well as scores on standardized tests as compared to suburban or rural school districts. During academic year 1997-98, Baltimore City had 17.6% of its students in special education. This figure is well above the national average of 12%. During the same time period, Baltimore City spent an average of $9,700 per pupil enrolled in special education. The city spent only $3,100 per pupil per year for those students not receiving any extra help in school. With almost 110,000 students in school, Baltimore would have nearly 1,936 students in special education, costing the city nearly $12,777,000 extra each year.(Figures based on Maryland School Performance Reports compiled by LEA:30 release 1.5, July 1999) The Abell Foundation, a Baltimore-based foundation, has dedicated itself to working to improve education in Baltimore and to identify interventions that show promise in helping to make Baltimore's motto a reality.

What To Test For? Learning-Related Visual Problems

Learning-related visual problems are defined as those problems or dysfunctions of the visual process that affect the child's ability to learn. These problems areas can be broken down into three types, which may be labeled nontechnically as tracking, teaming, and focusing.

The category of "tracking" problems for the purpose of this paper is defined as the inability to accurately and/or efficiently move through space and time the area of space the person selects from which the person is deriving meaning and directing action in. For example, in a sport such as tennis, the better players generally have a better ability to keep their "spotlight of attention" extremely close or nearly exactly centered on the ball as it travels in flight on a continuous basis. In the act of reading, the person must sequentially move his or her fixation point from place to place across the line of text. Different patterns of fixations, regressions, and return sweeps when looked at on a statistical basis or on a global basis reveal various scan patterns, each of which is characteristic of different types of reading and/or different levels of development in reading ability. These scan patterns are indicators of the degree to which a person has developed the ability to sequentially move his or her spotlight of attention across the page. Excessive amounts of head movement versus eye movement free of head and upper-body movement are measures of visual development level. Excessive numbers of fixations or regressions or an excessive number of regressions in proportion to the number of forward fixations are all indicators of a lack of development of the ability to extract information from the printed page. All of these would be considered as "tracking" problems. The most usual diagnostic codes used clinically would be the group of codes labeled ocular motor dysfunction (OMD), which includes the diagnoses OMD-Deficiencies of Saccadic Eye Movements (ICD-9-CM 379.57), OMD-Deficiencies of Pursuit Eye Movements (ICD-9-CM 379.58), and OMD-Abnormal Oculomotor Studies (ICD-9-CM 794.14).

The category of "teaming" problems for the purpose of this paper is defined as any difficulty or interference in using the bidirectional flow of data through each of the neurological channels (eyes to the brain and brain to the eyes) in a unified manner. This has been termed "binocularity." However, this term puts too much emphasis on the eyeballs, as in: "The two eyes are not teamed together." What is being hinted at here is a broader understanding of how the person builds his or her internal representation of reality. Hoffman[1] states that, "Vision is construction. Vision is not merely a matter of passive perception; it is an intelligent process of active construction. What you see is, invariably, what your visual intelligence constructs." When the person is effectively using the flow of data through both channels to and from the outside world in a seamless manner then their understanding, insights, and use of the space-time continuum that is the real world are greatly enhanced. (A single channel can be thought of as the connections from one eye to the brain and back again. Because we have two eyes and each is connected reciprocally with the brain there are two channels of flow. Alternately one could think functionally of the connections the brain has to each area of visual space. The right side of visual space goes to the left visual cortex through connections from the left side of the retina from each eye. In this way of organizing the view of channels, the channels would be functionally organized as linkages between the brain and the outside world, with each channel involving parts of each eye.) Interruptions in this seamless use of both channels of flow are clinically diagnosed as the following binocular dysfunctions: General Binocular Vision Dysfunction (ICD-9-CM 368.30), Suppression of Binocular Vision (ICD-9-CM 368.31), Fusion with Defective Stereopsis (ICD-9-CM 368.33), Convergence Insufficiency (ICD-9-CM 378.83), and Convergence Excess (ICD-9-CM 378.84) to name just a few.

The category of "focusing" problems for the purpose of this paper is defined as any difficulty in either (1) the selection of an area of space from which to derive meaning and direct action or (2) the inability to maintain visual attention at that location for as long as the person needs to sustain deriving meaning and direction of action at that place in space. These types of problems manifest clinically in one form as an inability to lock on to a target. Rather than fixate on an object directly, several attempts may be made in or around the location of the object. A person with this difficulty in achieving a lock-on of the spotlight of attention and of fixation displays behavior that is observed as high levels of distractibility and may be classified as having an attention problem such as attention deficit disorder with or without the hyperactivity.

The peripheral or magnocellular visual system is highly specialized as an alarm system and is excellent at detecting change in the environment and acts as an alarm system or threat indicator. If the person is unable to get a good central lock-on to the object of regard, these threat indicators may trigger forms of the primitive startle reflex, resulting in the person's attention being drawn off task, which may thus appear to be a fundamental attention problem. Unfortunately the formal diagnostic categories available to the profession of optometry do not fully address the manner in which visual attention is currently understood. It has become very difficult to tease out of attention models the exact degree to which visual process difficulties appear or are revealed as general problems of attention. In many instances the problems become absolutely intertwined so that it becomes impossible to delineate where the visual attention problem begins and ends and where the general attention problem begins and ends. It is not within the scope of license of optometry to make the diagnosis of attention deficit disorder (ADD) either with or without the hyperactive component. The formal diagnosis of Accommodative Dysfunction (ICD-9-CM 367.5) applies only to one very small subset of the overall issue of visual attention, which is being addressed by using the term "focusing." Focusing in this context refers to both the actual appreciation of clarity or lack thereof in the perception of our lighted world and to the focusing and channeling of overall visual attention to perform the tasks necessary to derive meaning and direct action accurately and efficiently.

First Steps: What Is the Prevalence of "These Problems in Baltimore?

Different research protocols may require vastly different resources, may have very different price tags to conduct, as well as expose the program to various types of critiques. In each design there will be trade-offs between what is affordable and what will give the best information upon which to extrapolate to larger populations. Questions that had to be answered all kept coming back to a core question: what is the prevalence of learning-related visual problems (LRVPs) in the population to be studied? The lower the prevalence the more schools that would need to be included to get the number of subjects and the number of matched controls in the study for significance to emerge from the data. The higher the prevalence of LRVPs, the fewer schools that would be needed for significance to emerge.

In general, the minimum number of subjects needed in a study provide data that can readily be extrapolated to larger populations has been established by those involved in statistics as 30. Estimates were needed to determine how many children should be included on the front end of the study to guarantee that at least 30 completed the program.

There were other circumstances that had to be considered in working to achieve N = 30. The treatment protocols would mirror that done in my private practice. The curriculum of vision therapy done in my practice is exactly that which is taught by the Baltimore Academy for Behavioral Optometry (BABO) for the treatment of LRVPs. The average length of treatment for LRVPs in private practice is from six to eight months. Abell Foundation representatives with work experience in the Baltimore City Public Schools warned me to expect major problems with attendance as well as with children moving in and out of specific schools. These problems could easily diminish the numbers in both the control and treatment groups once a study protocol was established and later as the study moved well into the execution phase. Thus, any protocol design would have to be robust enough to take into account these factors leading to potentially high dropout rates.

Visual Screening To Establish Prevalence

During academic year 1997-98, the Baltimore City Public School system had 112 elementary schools. Representatives of the Abell Foundation helped by selecting two schools that they had experience with in which visual screenings would be performed to collect the prevalence data needed to develop the research protocol that would be used in the full treatment program. The two schools selected, Hampstead Hill Elementary School and Westport Elementary School, were from two neighborhoods in Baltimore City that represented a cross section of the city. Both schools were in economically depressed areas of the city, one on the west side of the downtown area and one on the east side of the downtown area. One area had predominantly Caucasian children, the other had children who were predominantly African-American. Testing was done on all first- and third-graders present in these schools on the day of their respective screenings.

I was given the school scores for the prior three years on the Maryland School Performance Assessment Program (MSPAP) testing. This is a test given in the state of Maryland to assess the level of education at each school and is used as a measure of how well that school is performing its duties. No individual scores are obtained, only grouped scores to compare one school to another and each school against a minimum standard level. The lower the number the worse the children have assimilated what is being taught and/or can apply what they have learned to the test. Westport Elementary School had scores in the lowest rankings in the state at 2.8 in 1994, 3.5 in 1995, and 3.3 in 1996. Hampstead Hill ranked in the top 10% of the Baltimore City Public Schools but still had ratings of only 13.8 in 1994, 11.4 in 1995, and 15.9 in 1996.(Figures extracted from an article in the Baltimore Sun newspaper by Abell Foundation Staff in the fall of 1997.) (These numbers are out of a possible 100.)

The following is the screening battery, performed by optometric office staff including vision therapists. No optometrists were directly involved in the visual screening. Tests done included the New York State Optometric Association (NYSOA) King-Devic Saccadic Test, convergence near point (CNP) or near point of convergence (NPC), Randot Stereo Acuity, Keystone Visual Skills 4-Ball Test at both distance and near, 30-second +/- 2.00 flipper cycle testing, +1.50 diopter test at far point, and distance visual acuity. Table 1 shows the criteria used for each test to determine the presence or absence of a visual problem. The pass/fail criteria were the same for both age groups tested on all tests except for the NYSOA King Devic Saccadic Test, for which a longer time was allowed for the first-graders than the third-graders.

Table 1. Visual Screening Pass/Fail Criteria

Test	First-Grade Criteria	Third-Grade Criteria
NYSOA King-Devic Saccadic Test	> 150 sec	> 100 sec
CNP/NPC	>= 4 inches	>= 4 inches
Randot Stereo Acuity	> 50 sec of arc	> 50 sec of arc
Keystone 4-Ball Test Distance & Near	2 or 4 balls	2 or 4 balls
30-second +/- 2.00 Flipper Test	< 8 flips	< 8 flips
+1.50 Distance Test	20/20 or better VA	20/20 or better VA
Visual Acuity	Worse than 20/40	Worse than 20/40

Screening Results

A total of 129 students were tested at Hampstead Hill Elementary School, divided into 60 first-graders and 69 third-graders. A total of 136 students were tested a Westport Elementary School, divided into 79 first-graders and 57 third-graders.

Table 2. Visual Screening Data

Test	Failures (% of total)			
	Hampstead Hill First Grade (N=60)	Hampstead Hill Third Grade (N=69)	Westport First Grade (N=79)	Westport Third Grade (N=57)
NYSOA King-Devic Saccadic Test	34 (56.6%)	12 (17.4%)	55 (69.6%)	19 (33.3%)
CNP/NPC	9 (15%)	15 (21.7%)	14 (17.7%)	12 (21.0%)
Randot Stereo Acuity	23 (38.3%)	10 (14.5%)	29 (36.7%)	21 (36.8%)
Keystone 4-Ball Test Distance	23 (38.3%)	29 (42.0%)	30 (37.9%)	24 (42.1%)
Keystone 4-Ball Test Near	18 (30%)	17 (24.6%)	20 (25.3%)	22 (38.6%)
30-second +/- 2.00 Flipper Test	25 (41.6%)	14 (20.3%)	33 (41.8%)	22 (38.6%)
+1.50 Distance Test	8 (13.3%)	8 (11.6%)	8 (10.1%)	3 (5.3%)
Visual Acuity	0	0	0	0

How Many Were OK?

Of all children tested at Westport Elementary School, only 20 of 136, or 14.7%, did not fail any area of the screening. Of all children tested at Hampstead Hill Elementary School only 34 of the 129, or 26.47%, did not fail any area of the screening. Across both schools this means that 54 of the 265 children or just a mere 20.4% passed the entire screening battery.

Discussion of the Screening Data

Several things are interesting to note. In both schools the failure rates on the NYSOA King-Devic Saccadic test dropped from the first to the third grades. The score for failure in both instances was one standard deviation slower than the expected value for the age group being tested. This is a slightly looser standard than might be more formally used, which would often be two standard deviations below age expected. However, one standard deviation below was used here as a general indicator of problems in the overall population being tested. Additionally, the higher the N values are above 30, the more significant smaller differences become, allowing tighter standards. In both schools there were some exceptionally long times for a few of the first-graders on this test, because some of these children didn't know their numbers well enough or reliably enough to get through the test. Some did not even know the names of all 10 single-digit numbers.

The percentage of children who demonstrated a lack of ability to converge up to the four-inch standard on the CNP test increased in both schools as the children got older. The percentages were very similar in both schools, increasing from the low of 15% and 17.7% with receded CNPs in the first grade to 21.7%

and 21.0% in the third grades. A longitudinal study following the same group of children would be needed to detect significance in the emergence of these problems during the first few years of school. Lieberman[2] used the same criteria in the validation work on the NYSOA Screening Battery. With an N of 1963 students tested they found a failure rate of only 4.6%. Cooper and Duckman[3] found a median rate of 7% of the population with convergence insufficiency across a number of studies.

The Random Dot Stereo test used is the special Randot test (Stereo Optical, Inc. Chicago, Illinois, with both object and background done completely with random dot patterns. This test often shows lower measures of stereopsis than those tests with solid objects on random dot backgrounds or those stereo tests with solid objects in the absence of random dot backgrounds, such as Wirt Circles, which appear on the opposite side of the Stereo Fly. These more traditionally used tests have monocular clues to depth that may be used by the subject that are not present in the fully random dot test used in this screening. This may account for the higher than expected fail rate on the Randot Stereo Acuity test and may actually be more indicative of the teaming problems described above. Lieberman[2] used the Wirt Circles stereo acuity test as part of the NYSOA Screening Battery and their failure criteria was less than 60 seconds of arc. The test they used did not have finer samples below 40 seconds of arc. Despite this they still had a 16.6% failure rate on an N of 1979 subjects. Our rates, which were in the middle 30th percentile for three of the four groups tested, were significantly higher.

Upon review of the data, the number of failing responses on the 4-Ball Keystone Skills Test distance and near cards seems higher than expected. Some types of stereoscopes require different degrees of separation on the cards to measure orthophoria. Using a card designed for one stereoscope in one with a different separation may generate false-positive results. However, the stereoscope used for the screening was the Keystone Ophthalmic Telebinocular model 46C for which the cards were developed. Therefore those responses that had many children seeing either two or four balls–which indicates either suppression of binocular vision or a misalignment of the two channels–are not to be discounted and may indeed be an indicator of general teaming or binocularity problems in this population. Lieberman,[2] using the same criteria we did, found a 7.8% failure rate at distance with an N of 1973 and a failure rate of 10.6% at near with an N of 1971.

A rather high percentage of the children tested could not complete the minimum eight flips of the +2.00/-2.00 diopters binocular flippers in the 30 seconds. It is felt that this relates to their inability to shift attention efficiently from one location in space to another, particularly along the z-axis, which is toward and away from the self. Lieberman[2] used six flips in 30 seconds and he found a 37.0% failure rate in an N of 1969 subjects.

The +1.50 diopter distance test was used to screen for adverse hyperopia. Adverse hyperopia is defined as an amount of hyperopia, or farsightedness, which when left fully uncompensated for at near often is a major factor in an inability to sustain visual attention at near for long periods of time. The number of children with adverse hyperopia ranged from 5.3% to 13.3% in each of the four groups tested. Lieberman[2] used the same criteria and found a much higher failure rate of 30.6% based on an N of 1963 subjects.

The final finding was not fully unexpected. However, one would have expected out of a total of 265 children or 530 eyes that at least one channel in one child would be found to be incapable of reading at least 20/40 visual acuity. This was not so. Every child with each eye was able to read at least 20/40 in each condition. Therefore there were no high degrees of refractive conditions beyond the adverse hyperopia already mentioned above, nor was any amblyopia detected in this particular sampling.

Looked at as a whole, the data from the visual screenings demonstrated that there was a very high level of prevalence of tracking, teaming, and focusing difficulties in the populations tested. This was very significant in moving to phase 2 of the research program–the formal design of the testing and treatment protocols.

How Many Subjects?

The data collected from the screening showed that a very high percentage (approximately 80%) of the children in the Baltimore City Public Schools displayed evidence of LRVPs. The target minimum sample size of 30 in both the control and treatment groups would need to be higher to account for the expected drop-out rates. To strengthen the conclusion of the study, the target number of subjects in both the control and treatment groups was bumped to 50 children. Therefore, 75 students were to be selected for and provided with vision therapy. Over the length of the study, if one-third of each group were lost to follow-up then there would still be 50 in each of the groups. If the attrition in each group were greater, then the ability to extrapolate to the broader base of students in Baltimore City would be compromised. However, the study could have sustained as much as a 50% loss of subjects in each group and still have had more than the required 30 subjects in each to merit publication.

How Many Schools?

With the target sample data size set at 150 with 75 to be randomly assigned in each group, the next question to address was how many schools would be needed to satisfy these numbers. Six candidate schools were invited to a meeting at which the main concepts of the study were presented and what was expected of each school in terms of space and access to children was explained.

Of the six schools, four indicated strong desire to have their school selected as a site for the program. Site visits were arranged to each of these four schools to determine suitability of space for the testing and treatment phases of the program. Information was obtained that gave the total number of fourth-grade students enrolled at each school for the academic year of 1997-98. Additional data included the percent of the children in the third and the fifth grades at each school who had scored satisfactory on the MSPAP testing done in 1997. The final piece of data supplied was the percentage of children on the Free/Reduced Lunch Program, which could be considered a measure of the general economic status of the area. Neither of the two schools at which the screening had been done had been included on the school candidate list. Table 3 shows the candidate school profile.

Table 3. Candidate School Profile

School	Fourth-Grade Enrollment	MSPAP Reading, % Satisfactory, Third Grade	MSPAP Reading, % Satisfactory, Fifth Grade	Free/Reduced Lunch Program, % of enrollment
#254	192	5.2	6.9	84
#27	125	6	1.6	90
#215	139	10	15.6	61
#36	203	6.5	11.7	94
#95	120	12.3	6.2	91
#98	156	6.7	8	100

School #254 and school #27 decided after the meeting to withdraw their school from consideration. School #36 and school #98 had the required number of students to perform the entire program in a single school. If either of the other schools were chosen then at least two schools would have to be involved in the study to achieve the full size of the two groups as determined above.

There were rather strong pros and cons to working with one, two, or four schools. There were several benefits of doing the entire program in one school. By working with one school, only one set of equipment would need to be purchased and only one team of vision therapists would be required to conduct training and be monitored for quality control. Because the controls and treatment groups would be in the exact same environment, same school, same teachers, same curriculum, same neighborhoods, same socioeconomic profiles, etc., the controls would truly be as matched as possible with the treatment group. Thus, working all within one school had great appeal.

However, by working in a single school the potential existed for some problems as well. One such problem relates to the ability to make generalizations to other schools or other parts of the city regardless of how successful or not things looked at the one school chosen. Another great concern was whether an event that took place either at that school or in that community during the period of the study could greatly influence the measured effects of the treatment.

Another consideration was to use a single school as a treatment school and a second school as a matched control. The benefits of this would be that it would be very easy to keep the two groups apart to make sure that no transfer occurred during off time between the two groups. Potential problems of this would include the constant nagging suspicion, no matter how the numbers looked, of whether or not the two schools were truly matched in every respect. Even if the front-end data looked like the samples were the same, could it be said with any degree of certainty that every aspect that would have been controlled in a single school would be controlled to the same degree? I did not feel that this could be guaranteed. Additionally, it would be hard to keep the testing staff fully masked when they did the post-testing. Based on which school they went to, to perform the post-testing they would know which children were treatment children and which were control children. The staff could never be allowed to know that the protocols specified an entire school as a treatment group and the other as a control. It wouldn't take a tester too long to figure out which school they were testing, which could potential affect their post-testing results. I did not want there to be such an easy "give-away" to those doing the post-testing.

An additional protocol could have been developed that would work in up to four different schools at the same time. Could this assure more homogeneity by using two schools for treatment and two for control? Better yet, could half of the children in each of the four schools be randomly assigned to the treatment group and half assigned to the control group so that statistics could eventually be measured between groups in a single school and then among groups in different schools? Clearly this was the best choice. However, the implications were that four schools would have to be equipped with staff and equipment. Logistics of training four treatment teams and arranging for the testing at four separate sites would also have to be worked out. Quality control and supervision issues appeared overwhelming with this type of protocol, although it was recognized that it was potentially the best overall. Lastly, there were some challenges to think about in terms of the added levels of complexity that would be associated with the statistics of such a complex design.

The strongest plea for our services was coming from the largest of the four schools still in the running, school #36. When space for treatment at each of the other three schools was deemed to be inadequate and the rental of a temporary trailer for the vision therapy facilities at each of the other schools was factored in, school #36 was chosen as the single school in which to conduct phase 2 of the research, phase 1 having been the screening programs.

What Grade/Age Groups To Work With?

At this point another critical decision had to be made. What age group of students should be worked with? There were quite a few things that went into the selection that was made. I was given the impression by the foundation that within approximately two years they wanted to see some preliminary results that indicated that moneys were being spent on a worthwhile program. I did not know to what degree the problems were developmental in nature versus being influenced by other factors beyond the scope of what is seen in a typical cross section of private practices around the country that provide vision therapy services. In other words, were there factors that had not yet been encountered in the private practice setting that would alter the potential for improvement? If so, to what degree would these factors militate against the work showing benefits? If these other factors were present, to what degree would picking a specific age group maximize the potential to show an impact in two years? If the study showed benefits on this age group then additional funding might be granted later to investigate other age groups.

It was anticipated that the curriculum of treatment would mirror what I had been using in my private practice for many years and was being taught in the core courses by the Baltimore Academy for Behavioral Optometry (BABO) in its series of postgraduate clinical education for optometry. This same curriculum was responsible for a 73% improvement in reading speed with improved comprehension on higher grade-level demand reading passages in a study of 44 consecutive cases in my private optometric practice. This study used the OBER2 Eye Movement Recording Device before and after vision therapy to record eye movements and provided objective proof of the effectiveness of the treatment.[4] To what degree could the same levels of change be expected in an inner-city population and what age groups would show similar types of change?

If the problem in this population is purely a vision development problem then a graph of performance levels versus age would look similar to that shown in Figure 1.

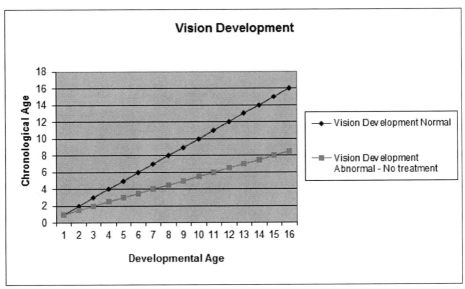

Figure 1. Normal versus abnormal vision development.

Figure 1 shows the developmental age plotted against the chronological age of two different groups. At the origin they are assumed to be equal. The normal group progresses one year of development for one year of life on earth. The abnormal group progresses a half year for each year of life on earth. The later in life one looks at the two groups, the further apart the two groups are from each other and the easier it is on the front end of a study to know for certain that the two groups are indeed different. For statistical significance to emerge one needs base numbers on performance testing to be at a level that expected differences and expected change as a result of an intervention could demonstrate such significance.

One could easily make the case that the problems would be relatively easy to identify and much easier to treat in the very young child. However, to demonstrate significance of a treatment modality it might take a very long time until such significance were to emerge.

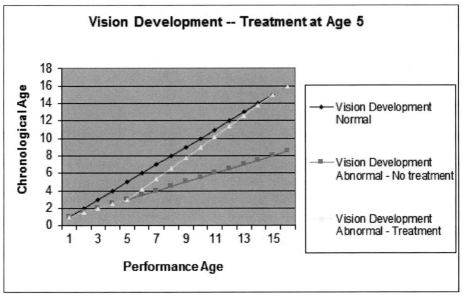

Figure 2. Vision development: treatment at age 5.

Figure 2 simulates what one might expect if treatment was given at age 5, the average age of a kindergartner, and the treatment group is plotted with an accelerated growth rate of 1.2 years' performance change for each year of life until they level out with the normal group at age 15. The untreated abnormal development group continues to make 0.5 year of improvement for each year of life. In this scenario it can be seen that a very significant change has occurred within the treatment group that will show its impact well down the line. However, at the end of year one, there is only a 0.6- year difference between the treatment and nontreatment groups and only a 1.2-year difference between the two groups at the end of two years. Unless the groups are observed for a much longer period, the evidence of significance, particularly if the performance numbers on the tests given have very low absolute values, may be difficult to establish.

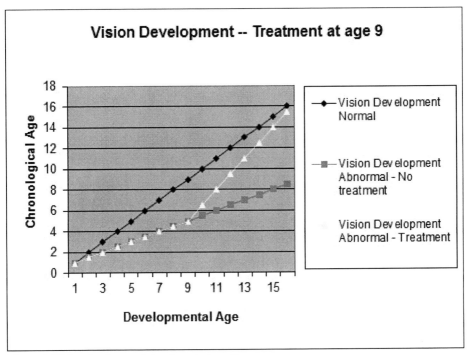

Figure 3. Vision development: treatment at age 9.

In Figure 3, the hypothetical treatment was begun at age nine or in fourth grade. The nontreatment group is again assumed to continue to develop at the rate of 0.5 year per one year of life. As of the time of treatment the treatment group is now assumed to develop at the rate of 1.5 years per year of life. Working with older children whose developmental lags could be more readily identified and to whom specific remediation offered, rather than giving mostly an across the board general treatment as would have to be designed for the five-year-old group, allows for the assumption that the benefits and the growth rate coming out of the treatment would be greater in the nine-year-old group than in the five-year-old group. Differences at the end of year one would now be 1.0 year of performance difference and would grow to a 2.0-year difference at the end of the second year after the conclusion of the treatment. This larger difference on top of a higher base of performance in absolute terms on the tests should reveal significance over a shorter period of time. In this case it takes seven years after treatment for nearly complete normalization whereas it took 10 years for the same to occur with the treatment begun at age five. This all assumes a high degree of linearity, which most likely could not be safely assumed. These graphs offer some insight into the thought process that led up to the selection of an older rather than a younger group for identification and treatment. If the study been established with a five- to seven- to 10-year follow-up from its inception, then younger age groups would have been selected because the intervention would have consisted of a simpler program that could have served more children for the same investment of time, effort, and energy.

Lastly, it was important to work with scales of performance, which were linear in nature and could allow the use of higher-order statistical analysis. Standardized testing was already being done regularly on these children. At a young age, many children might achieve a score of zero on a particular subtest or test. This score, although at an absolute floor, may not be linearly related to very low positive scores. This would introduce a degree of nonlinearity into the overall scheme. For example, on the screenings reported above, some children did not know their numbers and therefore could not perform on the NYSOA King-Devic Saccadic Test. It is one thing to say that they failed the screening. However, if one wanted to see reports on actual means and standard deviations for each of the groups, one would have to decide how to handle a child that failed because they didn't know their numbers. Would an artificially long time be assigned to that child to show clearly that they had failed? And after they learned their numbers and subsequently they did the test well and faster than the chosen slow time for them, would this demonstrate an actual improvement attributable to any specific treatment other than just learning their numbers? This conclusion could not be made in that instance. If these long times were used in the calculation of group means and group statistics, then the entire endeavor could be called into question.

For all the reasons cited above, fourth-graders were selected for this study. They would be available for two years in the elementary school. On most tests that were selected for them to take all children should be able to perform at or above the minimum scores on those tests so that either (1) no children would have to be eliminated from the study because their performance was too low to register on our measuring scales or (2) we would not have to manufacture specific scores for these low performers, which could affect the overall study.

Testing Begins

Funding for the research phase was approved mid-September of 1998 and by mid-October 1998, the testing phase of all fourth-graders at Harford Heights Elementary School (school #36) commenced. During that month the testing protocols were established and a statistician was consulted on the design of the entire program. During this phase three staff were hired as vision therapists for the research and their formal training began. Their training will be reported on later.

The following testing was done on all 178 children in the fourth grade. Some of these children were involved in special education for a portion of the day. None of the children in the full day dedicated special education classroom nor in the one classroom dedicated for emotionally and physically handicapped fourth-graders were included in the study. The 178 children were spread over nine separate classrooms. Fortunately, all nine classrooms were on a single floor around a central core, which included a library and a multipurpose room. A standard optometric testing lane with chair, stand, phoropter, projector, lensometer, trial lens set, and all hand instruments was set up in the health suite in another part of the school. All other testing was done in the centrally located library.

Testing done in the health suite included visual acuities distance and near; cover test distance and near; motility testing; convergence near point; color vision testing with Ishihara plates; the Special Randot Test; stress point retinoscopy; lensometry, if the child wore glasses; Worth 4-dot testing at distance, near, and at near through +/- 2.00 diopter flippers; and a complete analytical examination, which followed the guidelines published as Appendix A in Harris.[5]

Three optometrists were trained to perform the testing in a uniform manner. All had been active members of a Baltimore area study group for many years or had worked with me in my office and were fully familiar with the testing routines to be followed. None of these optometrists were involved in the training, the training of the vision therapists, or the analysis of the data in any way.

Testing done in the library area was broken down into three groups. One group was the Visagraph testing. Visagraph testing protocol will be explained in detail in the section that reports on the findings on the Visagraph. The second group of tests included the NYSOA King-Devic Saccadic Test, the Groffman Visual Tracing Test, the Wold Sentence Copy Test, parts I and II of the Jordan Left-Right Test, the Eye-Hand Coordination Sub-Test of the Developmental Test of Visual Perception II, the Gates Oral Reading Survey from the Handbook of Diagnostic Tests, and an oral history including a symptoms checklist. This section was called the visual performance testing area.

Dr. Ronald Berger, an optometrist from Columbia, Maryland, who was also a member of the Baltimore area study group, put together the third area of testing done in the library area. This drew heavily on the work of Swiss psychologist Jean Piaget and the work of Piagetian scholar Harry Wachs, a Maryland optometrist currently practicing in Washington, D.C. . Dr. Berger included tests of visual recall, visual transposition, auditory matching, auditory manipulation, visual–auditory integration, and learning motivation. These tests will be described in a separate paper; they are mentioned here only forcompleteness.

The children were given each part of the test on a different day so they would not become fatigued. No one section lasted more than 30 –minutes; the Visagraph station was the shortest test and the visual performance testing, including the oral symptoms checklist, took the longest time to complete. The testers in the library area were different staff than would be involved in the vision therapy.

The testing phase last approximately six weeks and was completed before Thanksgiving of 1998. A meeting was held with the statistician to decide the best way to separate the 178 children into treatment and control groups. In addition, test scores for the children on their national standardized testing were provided to us for the fall of 1998. These were the California Diagnostic Math Test and the California Diagnostic Reading Test by McGraw Hill.

Testing Results

The following are the results obtained on the 178 children as a whole. This data is reported here to give an idea of the total performance level of the entire fourth grade before the children were broken down into their respective groups.

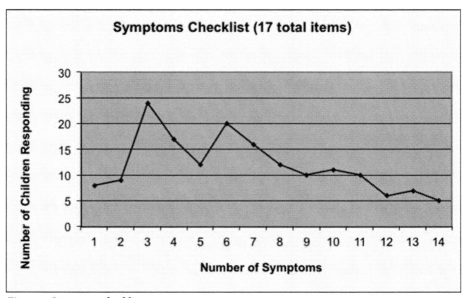

Figure 4. Symptoms checklist.

Symptoms Checklist

Complete data was obtained on 168 children on the symptoms checklist (Figure 4; Appendix A). The checklist was filled out by one of the testers; each question was asked of the child verbally.

Table 4. Top Five Complaints on the Symptoms Checklist

Headaches	84.3%
Uses finger to keep place with reading	78.1%
Eyes tired with reading/school work	70.8%
Loses place when reading	70.2%
Rubs eyes during the day	52.8%

Only one child did not respond to any of the items of the checklist with a "Yes" response. The average response was "Yes" to 6.53 items (SD= 3.53). Table 4 shows the top five complaints and the percentage of children responding to each.

Table 5. Distance Cover Test Results

Esotropia	4
Intermittent exotropia (>10 pd)	1
Significant esophoria (>10 pd)	4
Significant exophoria (>10 pd)	13
Orthophoria, low exophoria, low esophoria	149

The following findings are selected findings from the initial optometric analytical and chair tests (Table 5).

Of the 171 subjects on which this finding was recorded, four subjects were found to have constant esotropia and one subject was found to have an intermittent exotropia, which was more than 10 prism diopters. Four had an esophoria estimated to be more than 10 prism diopters, and 13 had exophoria estimated to be more than 10 prism diopters. Phorias were not neutralized with prisms but were estimated by the examiner based on the amount of movement noted during the alternate cover test.

Table 6. Near Cover Test Results

Esotropia	4
Exotropia	1
Low esophoria	4
Low exophoria	42
Moderate exophoria (>10 pd)	6
Orthophoria	106

At near the number of strabismics remained the same (Table 6). Those with esophorias at distance that were estimated to be more than 10 prism diopters still showed esophoria at near but the amount was now estimated, in all four cases, to be lower than 10 prism diopters. At distance 13 children showed exophorias greater than 10 prism diopters but at near this number was reduced to six. Forty-two children showed a low exophoria on near cover testing.

Convergence Near Point

Convergence Near Point (CNP) or Near Point of Convergence (NPC), as some call this test, was done using a Wolff Wand that was moved slowly from the patients' Harmon distance toward the bridge of their nose. The patient was asked to report the first instance when they noticed that the Wolff Wand no longer appeared to be single. The examiner also watched for any sign of either of the two eyes losing fixation on the Wolff Wand. The break point was recorded as the distance from the subject where either of these events occurred first. The average distance of the break point was found to be 1.82 inches (SD= 1.4 inches). Of the 171 students on whom data on this test was recorded only four students had CNPs of greater than four inches. An additional seven subjects had CNPs between three and four inches and 24 subjects had CNPs between two and three inches. Depending upon the criteria used for the diagnosis of convergence insufficiency, different levels of this condition would be diagnosed. Using a more conservative measure of four inches or greater would yield a very low percentage of only 2%. Using three inches or more would yield 11 subjects or 6% with convergence insufficiency and the strictest definition of two inches or more yields 35 subjects, or 20% of the population. Convergence insufficiency has a reported prevalence of from 1 to 25 percent in clinic population.[6-9] The median prevalence of convergence insufficiency in the general population is 7 percent, and it is similar for adults and children.[16]

Ocular Motilities

Ocular motility testing was done with a Wolff Wand. Separate pursuit and saccadic testing were not done. Rather than look at each of these components of ocular motility, the ability to keep the eyes on a moving target was tested as a whole. The Wolff Wand was moved in a pattern, which begins with a horizontal sweep, followed by a vertical sweep, then several diagonal sweeps. The movements then become circular and then include z-axis movements and variable speeds, and then start and stop as they cross the mid-line. Three things are rated, each on a scale of 1 to 4: the amount of head movement, the amount of supportive body movement, and the quality of the tracking (rated in terms of the percentage of time that the person is fixating the target directly).

The head movement scale is as follows:
1. No movement
2. Small
3. Moderate
4. All head movement

Of the 171 children on whom data is available on this test the average score for the amount of head movement was 1.59 (SD= 0.82) . Nine children were found to move their heads exclusively to track the Wolff Wand as it moved through space. When a target is tracked this way the person is essentially keeping the eyes steady in the head and using the supportive muscles of the neck and upper back to perform the tracking movement. Ten children were rated as a 3, which meant that a moderate amount of head movement was noted during the tracking of the target. This yields an incidence of 11% of the children (19/171) showing significant evidence of an ocular motor dysfunction based solely on the degree of head movement during a very simple tracking activity.

The amount of movement in the torso was found to be very small. A rating for the entire group of 1.00 would indicate that all subjects were rock-steady with their upper bodies. The actual rating for all 171 subjects was 1.11 (SD= 0.37). No children were given a rating of 4, which would have indicated that the tracking was being done exclusively using movements of the upper torso to track the moving target. Three children were given a rating of 3, which means that a significant amount of torso movement was noted during the testing. An additional 13 children were rated as having some movement in the upper body.

The accuracy of ocular motility was rated according to the following scale:
1. >95% accurate
2. <95% >75% of the time on target
3. <75% >50% of the time on target
4. <50% of the time on target

The total tracking score was rated for the 171 subjects at 1.71 (SD= 0.93). Eleven of the subjects were rated as a 4 and an additional 19 were rated as a 3 on the above scale. Thus, 30 of the 171 subjects, or 18%, were found to have accuracy of eye-tracking skills well below expected and well below that necessary to perform well in the educational environment.

Random Dot Stereo Acuity

The Special Random Dot Stereo Acuity test was administered. This test has both the object and the background done entirely with computer-generated random dot patterns. The test was given at a working distance of 16 inches with the patient's habitual lenses on or no lenses if the patient did not wear glasses or did not have their glasses with them.

Forty-three of the 177 children, or 24%, for whom data was collected on this test had stereo acuity that measured worse than 40 seconds of arc (Table 7). This number is much higher than has been seen in other testing of random samples of school-age children. Williams, in a study of children aged 7-11 found that stereo acuity levels improved as the children got older. In the study, which used the TNO stereo test they found that 52.7% of the seven-year-olds got 60 seconds of arc or better. By the age of nine 83.52% were now at this level and by age 11 84.8% had reached this level.

Ishihara color plates were used to screen for any color deficiencies. Of the 170 children for which data was collected only three children demonstrated any color vision problems.

Table 7. Randot Stereo Scores

Score (seconds of arc)	Number of Subjects
20	112
30	14
40	8
50	3
70	5
100	6
200	3
400	7
600	6
None seen*	13

*The child was not able to appreciate depth on even the grossest targets, which had 600 seconds of arc of stereo acuity.

Table 8. Values and Variation of the Subjective (OEP #7) Finding

Subjective Sphere	Value	Standard Deviation	Most Plus	Most Minus
OD Sphere	+0.53	+/- 1.36	+7.75	-7.75
OS Sphere	+0.58	+/- 1.36	+8.50	-8.50

Refractive Findings the following information shows the average refractive findings in the total group along with standard deviation and minimum and maximum refractive powers on the basic distance subjective. The finding as reported here is a binocular finding done after cylinder testing and binocular balance using a dissociation technique with a low amount of plus fog used for balancing. After balance is achieved, the examiner decreases plus binocularly or increases minus binocularly. The end point reported for the subjective refraction (OEP #7) is most plus or least minus to 20/20 visual acuity (Table 8).

The average values for the right and left eye refractive findings at just over one-half a diopter of plus is what would be expected in a random sample of the general population of young children who had yet to encounter lots of sustained near-point demands. The ranges for each eye are similar, with the left eye having a slightly wider overall range (17 diopters vs. 15.50 diopters.) and the standard deviations for each eye are the same at 1.36 diopters.

Prism Testing

An integral part of the analytical examination is the use of prisms at both distance and near. The patient is asked to look at a target, usually an eye chart, and prisms are symmetrically increased in front of both eyes simultaneously. The testing done by all optometrists in this study followed the same protocol. Base-out prisms were done first followed by base-in prisms. The prisms are increased until the patient reports seeing diplopia and then decreased slowly until they report seeing the images come back together. Table 9 gives the average responses to these tests on all subjects from whom data was obtainable. Some patients did not report seeing diplopia or did not report when they saw the images reconverge, even on a repeat of the test probe. This is why the number of subjects is not the same for all findings.

Table 9. Prism Duction Findings (Equilibrium)

Finding	Data	OEP Expecteds[6]	# of subjects
DV Base-out break	25.35	19	151
DV Base-out recovery	6.73	9	147
DV Base-in break	15.87	9	152
DV Base-in recovery	2.73	5	151
NV Base-out break	28.74	21	147
NV Base-out recovery	8.68	15	144
NV Base-in break	23.04	22	150
NV Base-in recovery	7.75	18	149

These findings are noteworthy in that all averages on the break points are higher than the OEP expecteds and all the recoveries are lower than the OEP expecteds. When large groups of findings are systematically higher on one side and lower on the other side, one possible explanation is that some of the members of the group are not good observers. By this is meant that either there is a longer than normal delay between the observance of an event and the reporting of an event. This could be due to systematic slowness of verbal response or overly fast moving of the prisms by the testers. It is also possible that the just noticeable difference in terms of detecting the diplopia or the refusion is wider than normal in these subjects. For example, the images may have doubled much earlier but they were not yet wide enough apart to trigger the person's report of diplopia. The two images had to be quite far apart before the person would report seeing diplopia. In this instance then the high number would be a false indicator for that finding and could not be construed to mean that the aspect of vision being measured by this test was indeed "normal." No attempt was made during the testing to tease out the exact reasons for these systematic differences in these findings versus the expected findings. The only way to do this would be to perform eye movement recordings at the same time as the base-in and base-out testing is being done and to analyze these recordings along with other brain wave recordings to assess when cognitive awareness of the events in question took place. This may yield interesting information but is beyond the scope of this paper.

Additional Test Results

One more set of findings from the analytical examination are the findings classically called Positive Relative Accommodation (PRA/OEP# 20) and Negative Relative Accommodation (NRA/OEP # 21). Table 10 summarizes this data and shows values here to be within the expected range again.

Table 10. Positive/Negative Relative Accommodation Results

Finding	Value in Diopters	Standard Deviation	OEP Expected
PRA # 20	- 2.57	+/- 1.47	- 2.25 to - 2.50
NRA # 21	+2.65	+/- 0.67	+1.75 to +2.00

The data in Table 11 is from some selected performance tests.

Table 11. Additional Performance Test Results

Test Name	Test Emphasis	Average Score	Fourth-Grade Norm
NYSOA - King Devic Saccadic Test	Eye movements for reading	82.91 sec +/- 19.51 sec	73.4 sec
Groffman Visual Tracing	Sustained visual attention and tracking for writing	13.3 points +/- 10.1 points	22 points
EH Subtest of DTVP-II	Eye hand coordination	8.41 yr +/- 1.82 yr	9 yr.
Wold Sentence Copy Test	Eye hand coordination and tracking	127.24 sec +/- 32.35 sec	144 sec
Gates Oral Reading Test	Oral reading without time pressure and without comprehension testing	Grade 4.62 +/- 1.06 years	Grade 4

The NYSOA King-Devic Saccadic Test[10-12] consists of three paragraphs of widely spaced numbers that must be called off as quickly as possible. Performance on this test relates directly to the eye movements associated with reading. The total time to complete all three paragraphs is reported in Table 12. The average for the entire group was 82.91 seconds (SD= 19.51 seconds). The norm for the average fourth grader is 73.4 seconds. Twenty-five children (14.0%) took longer to complete the test than the norm for the average 7-year-old, which is 100.89 seconds.

The Groffman Visual Tracing Test[13] consists of five intertwined lines that must be followed from beginning to end. Two factors are measured–speed and accuracy. No points are awarded if the child does not get to the correct end point. If they do get to the correct end point they are awarded more points for going faster and fewer points for going slower. The total points for all five lines are added together and this score is reported in Table 12. The maximum number of points that can be received on each trial is 10, with 50 points being the maximum for the entire test. This test relates to the eye monitoring skills necessary in those tasks where eye-hand coordination is essential, such as handwriting, and also involves sustained visual attention. The full group averaged 13.3 points (SD= 10.1 points). The norm for the average fourth grader is 22 points. On the Groffman Visual Tracing test, 70 subjects (39.3%) scored below the lowest norm on the test, which is 10 points for the average 7-year-old.

The Eye-Hand Coordination Sub-Test of the Developmental Test of Visual Perception II requires the child to draw a line with a pencil between progressively narrower corridors, some straight and wide, others narrow, some with turns, and others with curves. The more accurate the lines are drawn, the more points are awarded on each line segment of each trial. Each line segment is graded and the total points for all parts of the test are added up to derive a raw score. The raw score is then converted to an age-equivalent score using the tables in the back of the testing booklet. The entire group averaged 8.41 years (SD= 1.82 years). Fifty-seven children (32.0%) performed below the age of 7.5 years. The range of performance on this test was from 4.2 to 11.4 years of age.

The Wold Sentence Copy Test[4] consists of a sentence that must be copied as quickly as possible. The test was originally created as a vehicle to afford the tester an opportunity to observe postural and mechanical problems with copying tasks. Later, Wold applied normative data from other copying tasks to quantify how fast or slow the individual performed the copying task. The test group completed the test in an average time of 127.24 seconds (SD= 32.35 seconds). The norm for the average fourth-grader is 144 seconds. Twenty students took longer than the 166 seconds, which is the norm for the average second-grader.

The Oral Reading Diagnostic Test is from the Handbook of Diagnostic Tests for the Developmental Optometrist and is interpolated from the Gates-Mckillop Reading Diagnostic Test.[15] This oral reading test consists of seven paragraphs which when taken together are a single story about a boy, a dog, and a rat. Each paragraph is written at a progressively higher level of demand in terms of the decoding skills and/or the size of the sight word vocabulary required to read the passage successfully. The examiner listens carefully and marks on a recording sheet any errors made by the subject. For each paragraph a maximum of six points can be awarded. Based on the number of errors made for each paragraph a chart is consulted to determine how much of the maximum of six points per paragraph is awarded to the subject. The total scores for all seven paragraphs are totaled together to get the raw score for the test. (As soon as the subjects scores only one point or below on any given paragraph the test is terminated. Thus, a child may only read two or three paragraphs and a raw score of zero is assumed for all of the more difficult paragraphs. The total raw score then is converted using yet another table to a grade level or to an age score.)

This test does not investigate comprehension as part of the test and therefore is thought of as a decoding test only. Typically a child can decode words at a reading level higher than their comprehension level. The average child in the fourth grade at Harford Heights Elementary School was able to decode at the grade 4.62 level (SD= 1.06 grades). This is significant because it shows that these children are essentially at grade level in their ability to decode text. Only seven children were found to have decoding abilities below grade 3.0.

Visagraph

The 178 fourth-grade students were tested with the Visagraph, an infrared eye-movement recording device. A pair of goggles is placed on the child. The goggles are large enough to fit over any eyeglasses that a person might be wearing. The goggles are connected to an interface box, which in turn is connected to the serial port of a computer. In this case a Dell Inspiron 3500 running Windows 98 was used as the recording machine. Version 4 of the Visagraph program was used to collect and analyze the data.

The children were given a story to read silently. Testing is done with silent reading only. If a child starts to read the passage out loud the testing on that sample was discontinued and the directions to read silently were repeated and a new reading passage was chosen. There are seven to 10 different passages at each of the different reading levels available for use during the testing. The child reads from a printed test booklet. Some early versions of the eye-movement recording devices allowed for the reading passage to be read directly off a computer screen. All testing with the Visagraph for this study was done with the child reading from the printed texts in the booklet supplied with the device. Reading from a video display terminal (VDT) screen induces many additional variables into the recordings, which other researchers have documented. Because most of the reading done by the children in this school and in most inner-city public schools across the country is not done on a VDT, the standard printed reading samples supplied with the device by Taylor Associates, Inc. (Huntington, New York) were used.

All first sample recordings were used to acclimate the child to the testing situation and were not used in the data reported here. After reading the passage, the recording device was turned off and the child was asked 10 "Yes/No" questions to determine the level of comprehension. These questions are supplied in the test booklet. The same questions also come up on the computer screen after the recording has been completed. The questions are asked verbally of the patient and the examiners enters the subject's responses into the computer.

The mechanics of reading vary significantly as the demand level of passage reading changes. When the reading passage is more than one year below the person's instructional level, there are characteristic changes in the scan pattern used to move the eyes over the text. When the demand of the reading passage is more than one year above the person's instructional reading level and the child begins to get frustrated, there are often significant differences in the visual scan patterns. These variations can be very significant and could affect the data reported if the demand level is not controlled accurately in this type of testing.

Therefore, it is critical to have the reading passage be at the appropriate demand level for each subject. This is achieved by using comprehension level as the determining factor. The child was required to get at least 70% correct on the passage being read. If a passage was read and the child got less than 70% correct on the reading passage, then a new passage was read with the demand level lowered by one grade. The process was repeated until a demand level was found where the child got at least 70% correct on the reading passage. Fortunately with this sample of fourth-graders, the lowest-level readers were able to read with a minimum of 70% comprehension at the first-grade level. There were no children that could not read at the first grade-level. Stated positively, all children in the fourth grade at Harford Heights Elementary School were able to read with understanding at least at the first-grade level.

On the higher performance side, when a child got either 90% or 100% correct on the reading passage they were given a chance to try a harder reading passage. As long as they kept getting 90% or 100% correct on each passage, the child was given a new reading passage at a higher demand level. This was repeated until the highest level of demand was reached on which the child got a minimum of 70% comprehension. In this sample of fourth-grade children, only seven children were able to reach the fifth-grade level stories and still get the minimum of 70% comprehension. No children were able to reach the 70% minimum on a sixth-grade or higher level reading passage.

(First- through third-grade level demand stories are nine lines long. The middle seven lines on these passages have a total 50 words on them and the print is of the size normally seen in most early reading books [approximately Times Roman 16]. Fourth-grade cards and higher have 12 lines of text with a total of 100 words on the middle 10 lines. The print on these cards is smaller than for the first through third grade cards and is similar in size to the fonts used in most elementary and middle-school text books [approximately Times Roman 12.)

On the computerized reading testing done, the average reading level based on comprehension scores was grade 3.0 (SD= 0.96 years). Table 12 shows the distribution of children and the maximum grade level with at least 70% comprehension.

Table 12. Highest Grade Level Demand on Visagraph

Highest level attained with at least 70% comprehension	Number of children	Percentage of total
1	15	8.47%
2	33	18.64%
3	79	44.63%
4	43	24.29%
5	7	3.95%

Analysis of the Visagraph data also yields significant data relative to the mechanics of reading. By mechanics I am referring to the scan patterns, which are determined by the number of fixations, regressions, and return sweeps, as well as the average amount of time the person stops at each fixation during the reading act. A fixation is defined as occurring whenever the eyes remain at a fixed location on the text or the eyes are not in motion. A forward fixation is one that occurs as the person moves their eyes from left to right (assuming they are reading a left-to-right-read language such as English) within a single line of text. A regression or backward fixation occurs after the person has already had one or more fixation(s) on the same line of text at a position further to the right than where the eyes have just landed. Most of the time a person is not consciously aware of having made a regression. At times a reader may be aware of not understanding something and consciously going back to reread a section, a sentence, a passage, or a paragraph. This is entirely different from most regressions, which occur below conscious awareness in most readers.

Return sweeps are made at the end of each line of text. In theory they should be a single right-to-left movement from the location of the last fixation on the line to the starting point for reading on the next line. Often the return sweep in a beginning reader or a poor reader consists of a complex of eye movements in which most often there is a major movement from right to left, followed by a small correcting saccadic eye movement to get the eyes to the actual starting place for reading. Return sweep complexes are not normally analyzed separately. However, both the number of fixations and the number of regressions would tend to be higher in readers whose return sweep complexes have these small corrections on a routine basis.

Table 13 summarizes the mechanics of the full group of 178 fourth-graders tested.

Table 13. Visagraph Mechanics (178 subjects)

Mechanical Ability	Average Score	Grade Equivalent	Fourth- Grade Norm
Fixations/100 words	193.6	1.5	139
Regressions/100 words	43.5	1.8	31
Average Duration of Fixation (seconds)	0.33	1.0	0.27
Reading Speed (words per minute)	105.8	1.5	158

The full group averaged 193.6 fixations per 100 words, which is equivalent to a reader who is halfway through the first grade. These are many more fixations than are expected from the average fourth-grader, which is 139. This demonstrates that the children are stopping much more often with their eyes than the average fourth grader to read the passages. This can be thought of as adding to the demand of the reading task for comprehension as more separate pieces need to be assembled together from which the meaning is to be extracted.

The full group averaged 43.5 regressions per 100 words read, which is equivalent to a reader at grade 1.8 or nearing the end of first grade. Return sweeps are not counted in the number of regressions. This number includes only those backward fixations that occur within each line of text being read. The average fourth-grade reader is expected to have only 31 regressions per 100 words of text. The ratio of 43.5 regressions to 193.6 fixations shows that in this sample 22.4% of all fixations are regressions, which is exactly at the ratio of the regressions to fixations expected for the fourth-grader; 31 regressions to 139 fixations is 22.3%.

The average duration of fixation for the full group is 0.33 second, which is equal to that expected of a beginning first-grader. The norm expected for the average fourth-grader is 0.27 second. Although the difference of 0.06 second seems small, it is helpful to keep in mind that a college-level reader has an average duration of fixation of 0.24 second, which is only 0.03 second faster than the average fourth-grader. Thus the 0.06-second slowness in the average duration of fixation should be interpreted as significant.

Many things must occur during a fixation. The person must decode the word they are looking at. This acts as a key, which is used through associative memory to access the meaning of that word. The meaning or multiple meanings, depending on context, are integrated with what has come before in the reading and, typically, guesses based on knowledge of the syntax of the language being read and on contextual clues are made as to what is coming up. Additionally, and often as a parallel process in good readers, a process is functioning to preprocess to the right of fixation the spatial layout of the next area to be fixated so that the exact correct size saccadic eye movement can be programmed to be executed when needed. Good readers generally fixate one-third of the way into the next word. To do this accurately, because words are of varying length, there must be a preprocessing of the areas to the right of fixation to figure out where one-third the way into the next word is. Once the preprocessing is done the target area for landing with the next fixation can be plotted. All of these separate tasks may require very different amounts of time and can vary significantly during the reading. There is a huge variability in each fixation in terms of its length. The Visagraph data table only reports the average duration of fixation and does not give any sense of the degree of variability from one subject to another or from one passage to another within a single subject. However, viewing the actual raw recording data shows that some fixations may be as short as 175 milliseconds, whereas others may be 750 to 1000 milliseconds long. Often one sees these very long, single fixations occur at a time when the person stops taking in data from the printed text and goes internal to think about the data or to access other stored information they may have about the data being collected. A reinterpretation of the information already taken in may have to occur because something unexpected was encountered. When this occurs it is as if some readers go off-line for a second or more before resuming parsing of the text. Thus in some subjects the average duration of fixation could be longer because of either small increments of each fixation in time or the inclusion of several very long fixations. The Visagraph currently does not offer an automatic way to gain insights into this data.

Combining all factors on the children tested yields an average reading speed of 105.8 words per minute for the entire group, which is equivalent to the average child who is halfway through the first grade. The average reading speed for fourth-graders is 158 words per minute. Thus, the group of fourth-graders at Harford Heights Elementary School is reading 49.3% slower than average fourth-graders across the country.

Table 14 compares the actual reading speed for the group, broken down by reading level, against norms published by Taylor.[6] In general, the higher the level material that can be read and understood the faster the reading speed. Taylor's norms show that the average first-grader reads at about 80 words per minute and that by fifth grade the average reader is reading at 173 words per minute. I wanted to determine whether this type of relationship held in this sample.

Table 14. Reading Speed by Comprehension Level

Highest Level Attained with at Least 70% Comprehension	Number of Children	Taylor Reading Speed Norms	Reading Speed (words/min)
1	15	80	100.5 +/- 49.5
2	33	115	111.9 +/- 49.5
3	79	138	104.4 +/- 39.6
4	43	158	105.9 +/- 35.2
5	7	173	106.0 +/- 21.0

The table shows some very interesting information in that as the level of reading ability improved there were no commensurate increases in the average reading speed, as was expected. The 15 fourth-grade children who could only handle first-grade material as the highest level on which they could attain at least 70% of the comprehension test averaged 100.5 words per minute. The seven fourth-grade children who were able to handle fifth-grade material with at least 70% comprehension but who could not reach this same level of comprehension on sixth-grade material averaged just 106.0 words per minute. The average fifth-grade-level reader in Taylor's study read at 173 words per minute.

Speculating on why this might be the case leads to the following hypothesis, which is based on some observation. It appears that many teachers at this school may have concluded that the primary channel through which these children learn is not vision but audition. If these teacher are presenting material that they believe is important for the child to learn, they present the information verbally, usually in a group discussion format as opposed to the child being given a passage of text to read about the topic, followed by a group discussion. The end result is that there is actually a decrease in the amount of total time spent on reading for gathering information. A separate study would need to be done to address this concern and would involve charting the amount of time inner-city children spend at different tasks versus how suburban children spend their time during their academic day. My hypothesis is that significant variations exist that may explain some of the differences seen in these populations and may lead to recommended changes in the structure of the school day and in the manner of instruction.

Along the same lines I was interested in looking at the average duration of fixation in each of these groups to see how this finding varied or did not vary with reading demand level differences. These results are shown in Table 15.

Table 15. Average Duration of Fixation by Comprehension Level

Highest Level Attained with at Least 70% Comprehension	Number of Children	Taylor Average Duration of Fixation Norms	Average Duration of Fixation
1	15	0.33	0.33
2	33	0.30	0.31
3	79	0.28	0.34
4	43	0.27	0.34
5	7	0.27	0.33

As in the reading speed breakdown, the average duration of fixation does not follow the expected shortening with increased reading abilities in this population. The average duration of fixation is exactly the same for the 15 children whose highest level of reading on which they could get at least 70% comprehension was 0.33 second as it was for the seven children who could read and understand the fifth-grade-level stories.

One issue this raises is the impact that this may be having on the overall education of these children. It has been said that until fourth grade one learns to read and that from fourth grade on one uses reading to learn. If we assume that a significant portion of the child's school day is involved in using their own reading ability to learn from the printed page, then the children at Harford Heights Elementary School–and these children look representative of many other inner-city populations–are taking 50% longer on average to complete tasks than children with average skills in suburban areas. To compensate for this, the school day would have to be longer for the inner-city population simply to make up for the difference in the reading speeds between them and suburban schools. If, for example, the school day was six hours long and two hours of that day was found to involve children reading for information, then it would take the inner-city population three hours to complete what the suburban children were doing in two hours. Thus, to have the same intensity of educational experience would require that the inner-city schools only run a seven- hour day but also be certain that the entire extra time was devoted exclusively to reading for information tasks.

Note also that this does not at all compensate for the fact that the average reader in this school is one year behind in the demand level at which they can read and get information with good comprehension. This means that if the inner-city schools use fourth-grade texts that are written at the level that requires fourth-grade reading skills, then the textbooks are too difficult for the children to learn from. (I am unaware whether the issue of differing textbooks for inner-city versus suburban schools has been addressed.) Stated more plainly, in the subject of social studies, for example, is the fourth-grade child in the inner-city school given a social studies textbook that covers the fourth-grade curriculum on a fourth-grade intellectual basis but written for a third-grade-level reader? And is the child given 50% more time to read this special type of textbook than the average fourth-grader in a suburban school reading the material written at the fourth-grade level? To my knowledge this is not the case and to my knowledge this aspect of matching the needs of the population being served in both levels of demand and time required to complete the task has not been addressed. If I am correct, the inner-city child is given textbooks that match the curriculum needs, not the reading abilities of the child. Because of budgetary constraints, many of the textbooks used in the inner city are out of date. Over time, these discrepancies will lead to a wider and wider separation between the average inner-city child and the average child in suburbia, separate from all other influences such as socioeconomic, family structure, or cultural, which have been studied.

In the fall of 1998 the entire fourth grade was administered both the reading and math portions of the California Diagnostic Test. Table 16 gives the scores for these two tests on the entire fourth grade sample and the scores on the Visagraph grade level and the Gates Oral Reading Test.

Table 16. Standardized Tests Scores Compared with Visagraph and Gates

All Scores Reported as Grade Level	California Diagnostic Test Reading	California Diagnostic Test Math	Visagraph –Highest Grade Level with Comprehension	Gates Oral Reading Test
Score	3.23	3.44	2.95	4.62
SD	1.42	1.09	0.98	1.06
Variance	2.02	1.19	0.95	1.13
Minimum	0.00	0.00	1.0	2.2
Maximum	10.7	7.7	5.0	7.6

How Many Groups?

Another question to be answered was whether or not to have a two-group design (one control and one treatment) or a three-group design (one control, one treatment, one placebo treatment). There were many factors to consider. In many of the early meetings with schools, school administrators, and people within the Abell Foundation who had experience working in the schools I learned that one of the most difficult things we would have to overcome would be simply getting access to the children. We would not be allowed to take children at any time that conflicted with their "special" classes: physical education, library time, music, art, etc. We would not be allowed to take children during any time when tests were being administered. Initially it was stated that the morning time was a critical time, when reading instruction and actual reading assignments were assigned and that no pullouts, even by special education teachers, were to be allowed during this time. This later turned out not to be the case or we were able to get a special dispensation allowing us to work with children during this morning reading time. There were also space limitations for our program. In fact the vision therapy area was moved after the therapy part of the program had been going on after just two months. Should a three-group protocol have been selected a second area for therapy as well as additional staff and a placebo form of therapy would have had to be implemented.

Additionally, during the year prior to our starting the research, Sylvan Learning Centers had been subcontracted to provide certain tutoring services directly to students at this elementary school. Nearly 25% of the children in the fourth grade were already being taken out of the regular classroom for extra help through the Sylvan Learning Center. Information on which students were receiving this tutoring service was recorded in the children's records with the idea that on post hoc evaluations the Sylvan Learning Center work might be factored in as a potential placebo treatment group. By this I mean that certain subgroups of children were being brought out and given special attention on a regular basis. The intensity of the tutoring did not match the level of attention that the students were given in their vision therapy program because the vision therapy was done on a one-on-one basis whereas the Sylvan tutoring was done closer to a one-on-four staff-to-student ratio.

For all these reasons it was decided that two groups–one treatment group and one control group–would be randomly selected from the entire pool of fourth-graders at Harford Heights Elementary School.

Randomization

After consulting with Daniel Agley, who served as statistician for this program, nine performance variables were chosen for analysis of variance. These included the scores on the Wold Sentence Copy Test, the Groffman Visual Tracing

Test, the NYSOA King-Devic Saccadic Test, the Eye-Hand Coordination subtest of the Developmental Test of Visual Perception II, the Gates Oral Reading Test, the number of symptoms checked off on the symptoms checklist, the Berger Perception Tests, the Visagraph highest grade level with the minimum of 70% comprehension, and the reading subsection of the California Diagnostic Test.

A computer program was written to go through the entire database and to randomly assign 75 students to the treatment group;, everyone else was assigned to the control group. The program was run six times and the values of "C" for control or "T" for treatment were stored for each randomization. Variances were then calculated for each of the nine interest areas for each of the randomization runs. Dividing the larger variance by the smaller variance compared the variances for each of the nine interest areas. The closer the resultant was to 1.00 the more evenly matched the variances between groups would be. The randomization run with the lowest total variations of variances between groups was chosen. The actual means of each group were not compared, just the variances. Table 17 gives these scores on the two groups.

Table 17. Control Versus Treatment Group Scores

Interest Area	F-Score Comparing Variances
Visagraph Grade	1.0256
CDT Reading	1.0101
Wold Sentence Copy Test	1.3271
Groffman Visual Tracing Test	1.2167
Symptoms Checklist	1.2361
DTVP II Eye-Hand Subtest	1.0676
Berger Perception	1.2567
Gates Oral Reading	1.0026
NYSOA King-Devic Saccadic Test	1.0270

Training Therapy Staff

At the time the grant was approved in September of 1998, in parallel with the testing phase reported on above, three staff were hired and trained as vision therapy staff. They were put through an eight-week program to train them to perform the vision therapy. All three had teaching experience and one is the parent of a patient who had undergone vision therapy in my practice.

The chief vision therapist from my practice, Dennis Hoover, a Certified Optometric Vision Therapist, devoted most of his time to training the three therapists. Their training included some didactic work given by myself as well as hands-on work in each of the activities with each other under the supervision of Mr. Hoover. At about the three-week point each of the therapists began working with patients in my private practice under the direct supervision of my vision therapy staff.

Therapy Protocol

Over my 20 years of private practice and as a result of founding the Baltimore Academy for Behavioral Optometry (BABO), I had developed a curriculum of vision therapy for children with learning-related visual problems. This curriculum is based very much on the concepts of Robert Kraskin, as espoused in his series entitled, "VT in Action"[7] in which he recommends a broad-based treatment program that addresses providing the patient with the opportunity to have the necessary meaningful experiences to develop the skills and abilities necessary to meet the demands of the things that they wish to do in life. This philosophy does not assign specific therapy procedures or activities based on specific findings but rather provides a well-rounded curriculum to improve the person's vision. As a secondary effect one sees changes in the patient's findings.

The BABO Curriculum of Vision Therapy for Learning Related Vision Problems was adopted as the treatment protocol for this program. Because some of the more specialized equipment in the full BABO protocol was not available, the grid of activities was modified slightly to accommodate this. (See Appendix B for the grid of activities established for this treatment program. The grid shows only the names of the activities. Each activity procedure has been written up in detail and will be made available to anyone wishing to replicate the research protocol.)

This program is essentially the same program that in my private practice demonstrated a 73% improvement in reading speed with a 12% improvement in comprehension in a study done on 44 consecutive subjects as tested by the Visagraph.[1]

Homework?

An integral part of vision therapy as conducted in my practice as well as in most private practices around the country is to have the patient do homework on a regular basis. The protocol followed by most patients in my practice has them coming to the office for a weekly 50-minute visit. They are asked to perform 15 to 20 minutes of home practice on some of the activities they worked on in the office that week. They do not do homework on the day of their scheduled office appointment and they are given one day off during the week. Thus, I am looking for five days of practice between office visits. The typical office-centered vision therapy session has the patient working on five different activities for eight minutes each. This leaves 10 minutes at the end of the session for the parent to be taught how to do the homework with their child. A good bit of time is also spent during the session having the child demonstrate how they did an activity at home to be sure that it was done correctly before adding on the next level of an activity or before moving on to a new activity.

Avi Karni, an Israeli neurologist, makes the case very strongly for the need for regular practice sessions over an extended period of time to facilitate permanent changes in brain secondary to the learning and development that is taking place.[8] Karni states:

"Our observations suggest two stages in the acquisition of improved perception. A fast improvement, occurring early in training, can be induced by a limited number of trials, on a time scale of a few minutes or less… and then saturates, with performance remaining stable within the session and for up to 8 hours afterward. After this latent period, large and long-lasting improvements in performance were found. Performance continued to improve over days and was maximal after 5 to 10 consecutive training sessions spaced 1 to 3 days apart. Once a maximal level of performance was reached, most of the gain was retained over months and even years."

This supports the methodology followed by most successful therapy interventions in many fields. Short practice on a new procedure or activity in a control setting where performance changes rapidly during the session. This then must be followed by regular practice on the new activity at least five to 10 times with no more than a two-day break between practice sessions.

To be successful I wanted to be certain to include the appropriate amount of regular practice. Involving the parents and having the child be responsible for regular vision therapy homework would be one way to make this happen. Our symptoms checklist included asking about the home life of the child. We found that many were living with single parents, many were living with a single grandparent, and some were living with people to whom they were not related. A meeting for parents and guardians was set up and announced in fliers sent home with the children on two different days about a week apart. The meeting was held after school in the library, but only one parent attended the meeting. Because I doubted that a fourth-grader without parental support could be counted on to do the vision therapy homework on the basis needed to guarantee success, we used a different approach. The vision therapy was set up so that the children involved in active treatment would be seen on a one-on-one basis each school day for 30 minutes a day. During this time they were given four different activities, each of which was done for an average of 7.5 minutes. Because the therapists would not have to check on homework notes or to check whether the activity had been done correctly at home, nor would they have to assign new homework, nearly the entire 30-minute session was productive vision therapy. In a way, the children were receiving just as much actual working therapy in a 30-minute session in school as a private patient during a 50-minute session in a private practice setting.

Length of Treatment

The average LRVP patient following the BABO VT-II therapy curriculum will average nearly 32 treatment sessions when done in private practice. The in-school version of the therapy curriculum calls for a minimum of 70 treatment sessions. Because of holidays, school closings for teacher training and advancement, and absences for illness, it was hoped that the children would average four days of training per week. Thus the target of 70 treatment sessions could be completed in 17.5 weeks. Depending on when the extended breaks in the school calendar fell this could stretch to 6 months for the fastest children to complete the tasks. The therapists were given latitude to extend the amount of time on any particular activity if they believed the child would benefit from additional time on that particular activity. It was expected that the average child would need 15% longer than the minimum to complete the treatment protocol, some would need only the bare minimum, and some would require as much as 50% longer to complete the entire curriculum. Thus it was expected that some would finish in 70 sessions, and some might require as many as 105, with an average of approximately 80 sessions. Each child was given the same exact activities in the same exact sequence. The demand levels of the activities were adjusted by the therapist to the level necessitated by the patient's level of development. By making this adjustment each therapy activity could become a meaningful developmental experience for the child. (See Kraskin13 for more information on how to adjust difficulty levels of specific activities to meet the needs of specific patients.)

Schedules

The teachers, administration, and the master teacher for the fourth grade requested that we make up a schedule that had each child coming to their therapy session at a different time each day so that they didn't miss a full 6 months of a particular subject. A good bit of work went into setting up rotating schedules that still allowed every child to attend every one of their special classes (physical education, art, music, library, Sylvan Learning Center, reading tutor, speech, etc.). The vision therapy program began the week after Thanksgiving in the fall of 1998. A schedule was made up that took into account the amount of time the three vision therapists could work and the physical limitations of the vision therapy room. The schedule was found to accommodate 25 children. Three additional children were selected as alternates. Should any of the group of 25 be absent on a particular day, then the alternates would be called. This would decrease the amount of down time for the vision therapists and possibly allow several additional children to move through the process beyond the calculated maximum capacity of 25. An ambitious schedule was worked out over the academic years of fall 1998 to Spring 1999 and fall 1999 to spring 2000 to attempt to complete the three groups of 25 students chosen to be treated. This was not the ideal way to do this. The ideal way would be to have had all 75 in the treatment group getting their treatment beginning at the same time. However, space and time limitations set the maximum number of children that could be seen daily by three vision therapists working one-on-one to 25.

Stress-Relieving Lenses

Each member of the treatment group was given a pair of stress-relieving lenses to be kept at school and to be used during all sustained close work and desk work in the classroom. The analytical evaluations along with the results of the stress point retinoscopy were used to determine the appropriate level of plus that was prescribed for near point work. Each prescription was customized for that particular child. Prescribing principles as taught as part of the BABO Behavioral Vision Care course were followed. It is beyond the scope of this paper to go into the exact steps whereby the prescription was derived. However, it should be noted that a standard prescribing system was used that resulted in each child getting the lens that was appropriate for them. The lenses were all supplied in single-vision form. Generally speaking, no plus was given that was higher than the modified stress point retinoscopy lens and no lenses were given that were less plus than the #14B (fused cross cylinder at near). Embeddedness was used as a guide as to which cases would most benefit from lenses closer to the #14B or closer to the maximum modified stress point retinoscopy lens. Other factors taken into account include the equilibrium findings, the #20 (Positive Relative Accommodation), the #21 (Negative Relative Accommodation), the #7/7A distance subjective, and all phorias. Marchon and Marcolin (Garden City, New York) donated frames for use in the study and New City Optical, a division of Southern Optical, (Baltimore, Maryland) supplied the lenses and edging services free of charge.

There turned out to be many problems with the glasses. They were often broken, necessitating regular repair and replacement. Despite directions to keep the glasses in school, many children took the glasses home and then proceeded to lose them. Some teachers did not, on a regular basis, begin the day by giving the children their glasses. Often when they did give the glasses out their continued use during the day was not supported and they were not collected at the end of the day. The end result was that the effectiveness of the glasses as a potential aid was greatly reduced. Typically I see a difference in those children who use their stress-relieving lenses regularly during therapy. This usually results in therapy being more effective, reaching higher levels of cure in shorter periods of time than when the lenses were not an integral part of the treatment program.

The First Cohort Finishes

Toward the end of the 1998-99 school year, 16 children of the first group of 25 had completed the therapy program. Three of the 25 had left the school and the alternates had taken their place in the schedule but had not yet completed the protocol. Six of the 25 were still working through the protocol but because of either absences or slow progression through the protocol, they were not yet far enough along to be considered as having completed the program. For purposes of comparison 19 controls were selected based on gender and class. Children from the same classes as the 16 children in the treatment group were chosen at random and with the same ratio of gender mix for the purposes of getting a glimpse into how the study was progressing. This was done to see what changes were taking place and as a quality control measure. The summer would provide an opportunity to continue the training of the therapists to bring them to a new level of effectiveness and to improve the quality of the program.

Repeat testing with the Visagraph showed the following changes in treatment group 1 as compared with the matched subset of controls (Table 18).

Table 18. Visagraph Data (First Cohort – Spring 1999)

	Control (N=19)	Treatment (N=16)
Grade Level Change	+0.48 yr.	+1.22 yr.
Reading Speed Change (percentage)	-1.7% slower	+13.7% faster
Number of Fixations (percentage)	+3.9% increased	-20.8% decreased
Number of Regressions (percentage)	-15.0% decreased	-32.4% decreased

Approximately seven months had passed between the initial testing and this interim point. The control group had made 0.48 year improvement in the grade level material that they could read and understand at the 70% minimum level of comprehension. The 16 treatment subjects improved by 1.22 years the grade level material that they could read over the same seven-month period. The control subjects had essentially no change in their reading speed. (Based on the above discussion of reading speeds, which showed that across the board the fourth-graders, regardless of the grade level read with comprehension, averaged right around 100 words per minute, one would not have expected any significant change in the control group and none was noted.) The treatment subjects were found to have increased their reading speed by 13.7%. Although this difference seems significant compared with a 1.7% decrease in speed in the control group it fell far short of the 73% improvement in reading speed as was demonstrated when the vision therapy was done with private practice patients in my office.[4] The change in reading speed was achieved by a 20.8% decrease in the number of fixations, as compared with a 3.9% increase in number of fixations by the control group, and a 32.4% decrease in the number of regressions, as compared with a 15.0% decrease in the control group.

Table 19 shows changes in the same groups of children in some of the selected performance tests.

Table 19. Selected Performance Tests (First Cohort – Spring 1999)

	Control (N=19)	Treatment (N=16)
Wold Sentence Copy Test (time)	+ 1.6% increased	- 9.1% decreased
Wold Grade Level Change	- 2 months	+ 10.7 months
Groffman Visual Tracing (score)	+ 71.0%	+ 157.0%
Groffman Grade Level Change	+ 15 months	+ 28 months
NYSOA King Devic Saccadic Test (time)	- 14.6%	- 14.1%

On the Wold Sentence Copy Test the control group had an insignificant increase in the time to complete the test of 1.6%, which would mean that based on norms the control group regressed by two months in their speed of copying over the seven months since they had been tested in the fall of 1998. The treatment group decreased the amount of time to copy the sentence by 9.1%, which translates into a 10.7-month improvement over the same seven-month period.

On the Groffman Visual Tracing test both groups improved significantly. The control group made a 71.0% improvement in their raw score, which translated into a 15-month improvement in performance. The treatment group improved their raw score by 157%, which translates into a 28-month improvement in performance, nearly double the improvement made by the control group.

On the NYSOA King-Devic Saccadic Test both groups improved their time by nearly exactly the same amount.

Mid-Term Critique

Although several significant gains had been achieved, as can be seen, I felt that the research subjects should have improved more significantly. The possible reasons for the shortfall of improvement may include but are not limited to:

(1) The alteration of my in-office program, which normally takes an average of 8 months with weekly visits and daily homework being compressed to a daily in-school 70 to 105-treatment session program.

(2) The use of new trainees rather than seasoned vision therapists.

(3) The lack of understanding by the children of what the program was about, why they had been chosen to be involved and what benefits they personally would derive.

(4) The fact that specifics of the optometric and performance data of the children in the treatment program were withheld from the vision therapists.

(5) Poor compliance with the use of the stress-relieving lenses.

(6) The fact that, due to using a randomization process of all children, some children in the research group may not have had a significant need for the vision therapy.

(7) Failure to integrate or connect VT with classroom experiences.

Corrective Actions Instituted

During the summer between the completion of the first treatment group and the beginning of the second the following actions were taken to improve the quality of care that was being delivered.

(1) Additional comprehensive education for the therapists was given over the summer with additional hands-on work in my office under my direct supervision.

(2) Before beginning treatment the research subjects would meet with a vision therapist one-on-one so that the child could understand why they have been chosen to receive this service and how it would help them. The vision therapist would share with them what vision therapy is and what changes they may expect as a result of the work being done.

(3) The comprehensive testing record of each child was reviewed with the therapists before beginning treatment so that they knew exactly what each child's visual condition was before beginning vision therapy. Goals for each of the students on the therapy procedures were set, in the same manner as is done in my private practice.

(4) An orientation meeting was to be set up with all fifth-grade teachers before the beginning of the next school year. The purpose of this meeting was to fully inform the teachers of the purpose and value of the program.

(5) A positive reward for positive use of the glasses system of behavioral modification will be instituted. In unannounced classroom visits by therapists or Dr. Harris, children would be awarded pencils and other educational items for demonstrating use of the glasses.

(6) Some children needed extra time to master some of the foundation activities. The therapists were mistakenly under the impression that for the sake of the research and uniformity they had to move the child along anyway to keep to the time schedule. The fact that this was going on despite directions to the contrary did not surface until after a detailed quality control review of the records showed that every child was perfectly on schedule. This misinformation was cleared up so that the therapists fully understood that a particular child could stay with

Table 20. Standardized Reading Scores

	Reading Score in Grade Level		
	Control (N=69)	Treatment 1 (N=20)	Treatment 2 (N=27)
CDT Reading, Pretest	3.25	2.87	3.08
CTBS Reading Post-test	4.54	4.69	4.50
Net Change (years)	+1.29	+1.82 (p=. 137)	+1.42 (p=.701)

an activity until mastery of that activity was achieved to the level the therapist deemed necessary.

We Are Thrown a Curve!

A major concern about a single-school design versus a four-school design was that an event might occur in that school or in that neighborhood that would affect in a major way the outcome of the study. During the summer of 1999 several major changes took place at Harford Heights Elementary School. The school was deemed by the Baltimore City Board of Education to be too large to be administered properly by a single administration. During the summer, the school board divided the school into two separate schools. The physical structure of the school was not altered, rather the administration of the school and all accounting and business aspects of the school were cut in two: the kindergarten, first, and second grades were grouped into a single entity, and the third through the fifth grades were grouped into a second entity. A new principal was hired and administrative staff was brought in for the third through fifth grades. The prior administration was also changed somewhat and stayed with the kindergarten through the second grade.

Additionally, the contract that the school had with the Sylvan Learning Center was not renewed. Half of the fifth-grade teaching corps transferred to a different school, retired from teaching, or left the area. Two of the teaching positions were filled with just one week to go before school started, one was filled the first week of school, and the final position was not filled until two weeks into the new school term. Because of all these changes a meeting with the new principal was scheduled. The meeting originally scheduled for early August 1999 was rescheduled several times as other pressing business, which required urgent attention of the new school principal, took priority. Two weeks before the start of academic year 1999–2000 I met with the new principal. A representative of the Abell Foundation was present at this meeting. Our concern was that without the support of the new administration the study would have to be terminated. The Abell representative was present to help salvage the study should such objections come up. Fortunately we learned that the new principal had heard something about what we had done and that what she had heard was good. She was aware of the previous administration's commitment to the program and she stated that she would honor the agreement and that we could continue our work.

As a result of these changes and the late restaffing at the school, the meeting with the teachers, which had been planned to be a half-day meeting, took place for 45 minutes one afternoon the week before the beginning of school.

The Race to the Finish

The few children from the first treatment group who had not finished by the end of the prior year completed their treatment in September or early October. A new group of 30 more students from the original treatment group selection were started. Of the first cohort of 25 that had been started 20 completed the treatment and were still enrolled in the school in the early spring of 2000 when it was time to perform the post-treatment testing. Of the 30 who began the treatment in September and October of 1999, 27 completed the treatment and were still enrolled at the school in the spring of 2000. This brought to 47 the total number of subjects of the original 75 chosen by the randomization process, just three under the target of 50 students through the program.

In mid-March of 2000 we were notified that because the out-going fifth-graders would be taking the CTBS tests and the MSPAP in May, we would not have access to any of the children in the month of April as they prepared for the testing. It would take a full month for the testing team to complete the full testing regimen on the full control and treatment groups, so therapy had to end the last day of March 2000. The administration granted permission for the testing phase to continue during the month of April.

Of the original 178 children tested, 75 had been randomly selected for treatment. Of the 60 or so children to receive some vision therapy 47 children completed the program and were still enrolled at Harford Heights Elementary School in the spring of 2000. Of the 103 other children who were in the control group, 73 children were present for the perceptual/performance testing, 69 took the CTBS standardized tests, and 71 were present for the final Visagraph testing and served as controls. Some children were present on the days that the Visagraph was tested but were absent every one of the days that the perceptual/performance testing was done. This accounts for the differences in the numbers of subjects in the control group reported in some of the tables that follow.

Post-treatment Data

Table 20 compares the children's reading level scores. They took the California Diagnostic Test Reading and Math tests in the fall of 1998 as fourth-graders. In the spring of 2000, as fifth-graders, they took the CTBS diagnostic tests. Approximately 17 months elapsed between these two tests. It is unfortunate that the children were given two different standardized tests as it would have been best to compare their scores before and after on the same exact tests. Both tests are produced by the same testing service, but they are not the same test.

Table 21: Standardized Math Scores

	Math Score in Grade Equivalent		
	Control (N=69)	Treatment 1 (N=20)	Treatment 2 (N=27)
CDT Math	3.64	3.30	3.24
CTBS Math	4.48	4.71	4.36
Net Change (years)	+0.84	+1.41 (p=.007)	+1.12 (p=.118)

When the scores for the CTBS were received during the summer of 2000 two additional statisticians were consulted on how to compare the CDT Reading and CDT Math scores from the fall of 1998 to the CTBS scores on tests given in the spring of 2000. The best way to make the analysis on these would have been to compare the either the scaled scores for each subtest with each other or to use the normalized curve equivalent scores. Both of these types of scores were supplied for the CTBS test scores given in the spring of 2000. However, the only scores that were supplied for the CDT Math and the CDT Reading tests given in the fall of 1998 were the grade equivalent scores for each test for each child.

The Abell Foundation has funded a central database for all students in the Baltimore City Public Schools so that research programs such as this one can access information for studies from one central source. The CTBS scores are in this central database but the CDT Math and CDT Reading test scores are not. The responsible parties in control of the test scores for the Baltimore City Public Schools are not cooperating at the present time with the central statistical database project run by the Center for Social Organization of Schools at the Johns Hopkins University. The representatives of the Baltimore City Public Schools have stated that their concern for the privacy of the individual students' scores overrides the potential benefits that might derive from studies such as this. Therefore, the scaled scores or the normalized curve equivalent scores for the subtests on the CDT Math and CDT Reading are not currently available to me. The statisticians noted that a comparison of the means could be done on the grade equivalent scores and that should the scaled scores or normalized curve equivalent scores be made available in the future, more powerful statistics could be done.

Testing in this inner-city school over the past five years had shown that, on average, the children - were making only a half-year increase in their reading scores for each year they were in school beginning after the second grade. While in second grade, testing had shown that these children scored near the national norms for all second graders. From this point on, for every year in school, the children fell back a half-year behind average students across the country. Thus, despite the efforts to concentrate on reading, this school and many in Baltimore City were, from the second grade on, making only about 6 month's progress in reading achievement for each child in school.

At the time of the pretesting the students in the control group were at the beginning of the fourth grade and showed a 0.75-year deficit from where they should have scored. At post-testing the control group was at the end of the fifth grade ready to go into sixth grade. Now the discrepancy was just under 1.5 years, which reinforces the earlier observation of slower than normal growth on standardized tests for reading.

The control group made 1.29 years improvement in the 17 months. The first treatment group made 1.82 years improvement and the second treatment group made 1.42 years improvement in the same time period. The scores for treatment group 1 are approaching significance, whereas those for group 2 show no significant change over the control group. The mean starting reading levels for each of these groups is not the same. Treatment group 1 started below each of the other two groups and finished with the highest level. The variances of the control and treatment group were matched before the testing. However, only 47 of the 75 treatment subjects were left and 69 of the 103 control subjects were left. The variances in the beginning scores and the means in these scores may now not be matched as they were before the dropouts over the 17-month period. There was no way to control for these losses and it was hoped that the random loss of some controls and some treatment subjects would not skew the beginning sets of data too much. The various measures of reading will be contrasted and unified into a continuum of reading later in this paper.

The control group made 0.84 year improvement in the 17 months in the area of mathematical abilities as opposed to 1.41 years in treatment group 1 and 1.12 years in treatment group 2 (Table 21). Treatment group 1 scores show highly significant changes beyond the .01 level. The scores for treatment group 2 approach significance. Many of the areas that vision therapy addresses directly affect spatial thinking, visual thinking, and visual problem-solving involving time and space relationships, which are the foundation on which mathematics is based. What begins to emerge from looking at the two treatment groups over time is that the first treatment group, having completed their therapy in the spring of 1999, had nearly one year of using their new skills in the classroom to facilitate the generalization of their new-found skills into higher-level testing such as the CTBS standardized tests. The groups will be tracked over time using the central database system. The hypothesis for scores over the next year in both math and reading would be that the control groups would continue to make slow progress– less than one year of progress for each year in school. Treatment group 2 should make a significant jump in this next year in all areas. Over the next few years both treatment groups should then continue to progress at or slightly better than the rate of one year growth in scores for each year remaining in the school system. Should this continue then the true merits of the intervention will be demonstrated so as to leave no doubt of the potential benefits of such a program.

Eye Movements and Reading

Table 22 shows the average in each group of the highest reading comprehension levels attainable with a minimum of 70% on the comprehension test, as tested using the infrared eye-movement recording device, the Visagraph.

Table 22. Visagraph Reading Grade Level Improvement

	Highest Grade Level Attainable with Minimum 70% Comprehension		
	Control (N=71)	Treatment 1 (N=20)	Treatment 2 (N=27)
Visagraph Grade Before	2.83	3.30	3.00
Visagraph Grade After	4.08	5.70	5.11
Net Change (years)	+1.25	+2.40 (p=.004)	+2.11 (p=.015)

The control group made a 1.25-year improvement in the 17 months of the study. Treatment group 1 made a 2.40-year improvement in the same time and treatment group 2 made a 2.11-year improvement. Both groups showed highly significant changes. Treatment group 1 would have closed almost entirely the gap in reading level scores between their performance and the level that at which they should be reading by the time they enter the sixth grade. It is anticipated that treatment group 2 only needs some additional time and additional practice using their new-found tools and skills in reading to fully close the gap as well over the next six to 12 months.

Table 23 compares reading speeds before and after treatment, based on the highest level reading passage on which students could achieve at least 70% comprehension both before and after treatment. This means that on average the children in the control group were being tested on 1.25 year's more difficult reading passages and those in the treatment groups on a more than 2-year increase in the difficulty of the passage read.

Table 23. Visagraph Reading Speed on Highest Demand Level

	Tested at Maximum Reading, Post-treatment (words per minute)		
	Control (N=71)	Treatment 1 (N=20)	Treatment 2 (N=27)
Reading Speed Before	112.37	107.75	97.81
Reading Speed After	124.11	106.85	129.96
Net Change (grade equivalent)	+11.74 (+0.48)	-0.9 (p=.378) (no change)	+31.82 (p=.106) (+1.17)

The control group improved their reading speed by 11.74 words per minute over the 17-month period. Based on the Taylor norms the average fourth-grade reader should be reading at 158 words per minute, at 173 words per minute by fifth grade, and at 185 words per minute by sixth grade, which these children were about to enter. Extrapolating from the norms, the control group moved

Table 25. Visagraph Reading Speed (Demand-Controlled). Students were tested at the same reading level post-test as pretest.

	Words per Minute		
	Control (N=71)	**Treatment 1 (N=20)**	**Treatment 2 (N=27)**
Reading Speed Before	112.37 (1.91)	107.75 (1.79)	97.81 (1.48)
Reading Speed After	128.17 (2.53)	131.30 (2.71)	139.41 (3.05)
Net Change (Grade Equivalent)	+15.80 (+0.62)	+23.55 (p=.577) (+0.92)	+41.60 (p=.039) (+1.57)

from grade equivalent (GE) score of grade 1.91 to grade 2.39, or 0.48 year change in 17 months. Treatment group 1, which finished its vision therapy in May 1999, showed an actual slowing of just less than one word per minute. Treatment group 2, which had just finished their vision therapy, had made 31.82 words per minute improvement. Their GE scores improved from a grade of 1.48 to 2.65, or 1.17 year change in 17 months.

The lack of speed change at this time in treatment group 1 on their 2.40-years more difficult reading passage is a bit puzzling. The final phase of the vision therapy uses a computer-based reading scan drill program, ReadFast, to train better eye movements. It does this by using a moving window, which parses the text to be read from left to right, showing about two to two-and-a-half words at a time. The speed of the window movement is controlled and is generally set from 10 to 20 words per minute faster than the person is currently comfortable reading. This helps to pace the person during reading and to stop them from making regressions. Because the window only shows the current fixation point and to the right of that, regressions are futile because they would be made to a blank zone on the computer screen.

The differences between the two treatment groups could be explained in several different ways. The first would be that the speed improvement seen directly after intense work with the ReadFast program is when reading speeds reach their maximum and that over time there is a rolling back of the reading speed to the former habitual speed.

A second explanation might be that many of the individual members of treatment group 1 had just recently jumped another level in the demand reading level at which they were able to read. For example, one of the subjects in this group began reading at 167 words per minute on a second-grade-level card. At the end of the treatment this child was now able to handle a junior high school-level reading card. However, this child's reading speed had now dropped to 116 words per minute. I am certain that most teachers and parents would rather have the child working at a much higher grade level even if they had to slow down their reading speed to achieve the increase in difficulty level.

Of the 20 children in treatment group 1, eight of the children read slower. Only two of the 20 children were not able to handle passages with any greater difficulty. All of the other children were able to read more difficult stories. (Above the sixth-grade level of difficulty the reading samples for the Visagraph have only two reading levels: junior high school and high school/college. Six of the eight children in this group were now able to read at the junior high school level of difficulty. These cards actually cover the spread from the traditional seventh-grade to ninth-grade levels of difficulty and most likely should have been counted in the statistics for maximum reading level as an average demand of eighth grade. However, they were counted as seventh-grade-level stories to keep the scales linear. This resulted in an underestimation or under-reporting of the increase in grade level difficulty handled, as reported above. Not only were six of the eight making this jump into the junior high school-level stories, but also all but two were making a three-year or more jump in demand level as well, even counting the junior high school-level stories at a grade value of 7.0. Six of 20 subjects (30%) in treatment group 1 and five of 27 subjects (18.5%) in treatment group 2 had advanced to the junior high school level. Only three of 71 control students (4.2%) advanced to this level.

Table 24 shows the grade level improvements now with the junior high school-level cards assigned a value of 8.0 for all subjects who successfully read this level story with a minimum level of 70% comprehension.

Table 24. Visagraph Reading Grade Level Improvement (with Junior High School = 8.0 Modification)

| | Highest Grade Level Attainable with Minimum 70% Comprehension | | |
	Control (N=71)	Treatment 1 (N=20)	Treatment 2 (N=27)
Visagraph Grade Before	2.83	3.30	3.00
Visagraph Grade After	4.13	6.00	5.30
Net Change (years)	+1.30	+2.70 (p=.001)	+2.30 (p=.009)

As a result of the change the spread between the control and treatment groups has increased and the measures of significance on a one-way analysis of variance has also increased for each treatment group.

A combination of both of these effects may also be in play. The only way to know for sure would be to watch groups of children closely as they improve in reading ability to see how comprehension levels and reading speeds interplay. The hypothesis is that as the child jumps to a new level of demand competency first there is a loss in speed, which rebounds over time as the child automates the skill at the new higher level. This would plateau for a period of time and then the cycle would continue.

A third explanation might be that the therapists put more emphasis on those activities that would foster greater speed changes with treatment group 2 than with treatment group 1. The therapy staff was extensively retrained during the summer between the times that treatment group 1 finished their treatment and treatment group 2 began treatment. However, this explanation would tend to be refuted by the fact that in the spring of 1999, 16 members of treatment group 1 showed a 13.7% increase in speed versus 19 members of the control group, who showed a 1.7% slowing of their reading speed. Thus, at one point, soon after the completion of the treatment phase, there was a speed increase. However, this was measured on the same level reading passage. This will be discussed more in the Discussion section.

I wanted to remove the grade level differential as a factor in comparing reading speeds before and after testing. Table 25 represents this reading-level-free comparison. To compile these data the children were given a reading passage on the post-test that matched the highest reading level they attained at the pretest session. Thus, if the highest level a child could read at and still get at least 70% correct on the comprehension in the pretest was fourth grade, then they were given a fourth-grade text at the post-test, even if they could now read on the junior high school grade level with comprehension greater than or equal to 70%.

With the reading level kept constant the control group made a GE change of from grade 1.91 to grade 2.52 or a 0.61-year improvement. The first treatment group made a GE change of from grade 1.79 to grade 2.71 or a 0.92-year improvement. The second treatment group made a GE change of from grade 1.48 to grade 3.05 or a 1.57-year improvement. This showed significance at the .05 level (p=0.039).

Selected Performance Tests

Table 26 reports on the differences in the NYSOA King-Devic Saccadic Test before and after the treatment. Four subjects from treatment group 2 were not present in school when this portion of the testing was done.

Table 26. NYSOA King-Devic Saccadic Test

| | Seconds to Complete All 3 Samples (Age in Years) | | |
	Control (N=73)	Treatment 1 (N=20)	Treatment 2 (N=23)
Before	80.60 (7.94)	84.68 (7.74)	78.48 (8.11)
After	61.11 (10.63)	59.29 (10.79)	59.52 (10.77)
Net Change	-19.49 (+2.69)	-25.39 (p=.209) (+3.05)	-18.96 (p=.963) (+2.66)

In each group the average times got faster and a net decrease in time to call off the numbers was noted (Table 27). The control group pared 19.49 seconds from their time to shift from a score equivalent to that of the average 8.0-year-old to that of the average 10.6-year-old. The ending score for all three groups is within a second of each other. Treatment group 1 made a bigger net change, but that may have been because they started at a lower level of performance. These differences were not significant.

Table 27. Groffman Visual Tracing

	Points Scored (Grade Equivalent)		
	Control (N=73)	Treatment 1 (N=20)	Treatment 2 (N=23)
Before	13.23 (7.46)	9.40 (6.94)	13.57 (7.51)
After	19.04 (8.41)	22.60 (9.15)	19.57 (8.51)
Net Change	+5.81 (+0.95)	+13.20 (p=.024) (+2.21)	+6.00 (p=.949) (+1.00)

Both the control group and treatment group 2 made very similar changes of 5.81 and 6.00 points, respectively, over the 17-month time of the project, which correspond to 0.95 and 1.00 year change, respectively. Their scores moved them from approximately a 7.5-year-old performance level to an 8.5-year-old performance level. Treatment group 1, however, moved from a 6.94-year-old performance level to a 9.15-year-old performance level. This was significant to the .05 level (p=0.024).

Changes in eye-hand coordination are summarized in Table 28.

Table 28. Eye-Hand Coordination Sub-Test of the Developmental Test of Visual Perception II

	Age Score		
	Control (N=73)	Treatment 1 (N=20)	Treatment 2 (N=23)
Before	8.17	8.14	8.47
After	9.21	9.55	9.92
Net Change	+1.04	+1.41 (p=.518)	+1.45 (p=.480)

The net change in the ability in both treatment groups showed an improvement in the actual score but these changes did not approach significance. The control group made 1.04-years improvement in the 17 months of the program, whereas the treatment groups made 1.41 and 1.45 years of improvement.

The results from the Gates Oral Reading Survey are shown in Table 29.

Table 29. Gates Oral Reading Survey

	Grade		
	Control (N=73)	Treatment 1 (N=20)	Treatment 2 (N=23)
Before	4.49	4.72	4.47
After	6.28	6.56	6.22
Net Change	+1.79	+1.84 (p=.813)	+1.75 (p=.862)

The reading survey results for the three groups are virtually indistinguishable from one another. There appears to be no difference in the children's ability to decode what they read. On average the entire group has the ability to decode at or slightly above their current grade placement. Certainly mastery of reading at the same level for comprehension is not at the same level and all measures of the mechanics of reading as measured by the Visagraph are much below these levels.

At the time of this writing much additional raw data remains that has not been given the attention it merits. Much of this is the data from the analytical examination as well as the other more "pure" optometric tests such as visual acuity, ocular motility, stereo acuity, near point retinoscopy, accommodative ranges, equilibrium findings, phoria measures, plus acceptance findings, cover testing, and more. Attention in reporting data has been slanted toward "performance" testing and/or standardized testing, as this is the area that the public is most concerned with. This represents the unmet needs of the population that the profession of optometry serves through the treatment modality vision therapy or visual training. Regardless of what changes occurred with the specific optometric findings, those concerned (the Abell Foundation, the parents of the children with LRVPs everywhere, teachers of children with LRVPs, and administrators of schools with children with LRVPs) were looking for changes in performance in the classroom and on standardized tests. Making a difference in these areas of performance will lead to continuance and future expansion of these types of programs.

Discussion

Reading performance on a standardized test requires the integration of all aspects of reading skills into the ability to get information from written material and to use that information to answer questions and to do so over a sustained period of time. When "reading" is investigated, few researchers report on the spectrum or continuum of reading abilities and scores, which correlate to the specific aspects of the reading process the tests are investigating. Attempting to quantify reading ability into a single number or a single score cannot begin to describe a child's strengths or weaknesses or to communicate the degree to which that same child can efficiently and effectively derive meaning from the printed page and put that information to use. The following is an attempt to give the reader a view of how "reading" has been investigated in this research.

The Gates Oral Reading Survey probes specifically into to what degree the child has broken the code of being able to say the words from the written paper. It is a decoding test only. This test typically yields the highest "reading level" of any reading test because it does not involve comprehension and is not a test that asks for performance to be sustained over any great period of time. The groups on the Gates Oral Reading Survey are all essentially the same, being somewhere in the middle of fourth grade at the beginning of the testing period and at the beginning to middle of sixth grade at the end of the program. There were no significant differences between the degree of change or the beginning or ending points. The test measures reading at the basic ability level of decoding only.

As stated before, when Visagraph recordings are made, comprehension is an integral part of the testing. A minimum of 70% on the comprehension test is required and reading demand levels are adjusted up and down until the appropriate demand level has been found. It is important to note that on reading passages below the fourth grade the passages are nine lines long and analysis is done on the middle seven lines, which average 50 words, and that all passages of fourth-grade-level difficulty and higher are 12 lines long and analysis is done on the middle 10 lines, which average 100 words. This test is more involved than the Gates Oral Reading Survey because it incorporates comprehension while measuring mechanical aspects of reading at the same time. When the Visagraph is recorded, the subject is aware that their reading speed is a part of the test. They are told to read for comprehension and they have to answer questions on what they read. They are not told directly that we are measuring their reading speed but they are told that their eye movements are being recorded into the computer. This causes some to be a bit more stressed during a formal recording than if they had been asked to read the story to themselves by just holding the card without the goggles on and without the computer being nearby.

It is important to note that the Visagraph test is very short in duration. For a reader doing a third-grade passage at 100 words per minute the total time to read the passage may be just 35 to 45 seconds. For the readers of the longer stories, the total time to read the entire 12 lines, which contain more than 100 words, may run from 70 to 85 seconds. Thus, those who have not yet fully integrated these new skills may perform well on a short-burst sprint like the Visagraph but have not yet generalized or integrated these skills and abilities such that they can perform at that level for the sustained periods of time, which is precisely what standardized testing requires.

Retesting at the end of the program was done at two different demand levels. In one instance testing was done at the same demand level that the children had read at during the pretreatment testing. The second was to test the child at the highest reading level they could understand at the 70% minimum comprehension level. It is known that as the demand level of the reading passage changes for a single reader, very large changes in reading speeds can be made. For example, if a person is reading a passage two years below their instructional level they can breeze through it very quickly with little effort. Their speed drops a bit when they are at their instructional level. When given something that is too hard, most people at first drop their speed significantly. Once in a while when a person perceives a passage to be just too hard they may give up or move into "flight." They don't actually quit or leave the situation physically; they continue to work on the task but their commitment in effort, energy, and resources drops significantly. At that time one may observe that any outward appearance that the person was concentrating is now gone. They back away from the text; tension is gone from the face and the posture, etc. At that point the reading speed usually increases dramatically. They have switched from "reading" to "skimming." When asked if they read the passage they will say, "Yes," but in fact about all they have done is pass their eyes over the text with little effort and even less comprehension. Therefore a one- or two-year level change on the demand can greatly affect the speed measures. So, one of the post-test reading passages was done at the previous demand level so that speeds could be directly compared. We believed this would maximize the speed differences and demand would be factored out.

The second set of data looked at the new maximum level of difficulty that the child could handle as a result of the treatment. What emerged from our data here and what has been seen in my general practice is the following. A vision therapy patient is able to shift up to harder difficulty levels rather early in the vision therapy process. The mechanics of reading may appear to regress during the initial phase of working on the higher demand material. Most teachers and parents are very happy that the child is handling more difficult material and few parents and teacher use stop watches to determine how quickly their children are reading. One would have to spend a good deal of time with a child to be able to detect 30% or 40% differences in reading speeds when a child is reading silently.

Many parents and teachers do notice changes in reading performance early in therapy. The primary way they become aware of this is through oral reading. What they typically detect are cadence differences in the oral reading. The child who is developing and learning better tracking, eye teaming (binocular), and focusing of visual attention skills typically can more quickly and more smoothly decode the words in front of him and recite them in a more connected manner. The Gates Oral Reading Survey helps us to see the reality, which is that the actual decoding ability is not really enhanced; rather, the system is working more efficiently and smoothly and therefore those who work with the child perceive there to be an improvement in reading when in reality the decoding skills are roughly unchanged.

Over time the child does begin to understand more difficult reading material. This does not happen because the vision therapy has increased his intellect nor because there has been a significant change in his reading ability. Rather, the change in the child's ability to derive meaning from the printed page has been enhanced very significantly because the process of vision has been improved by working on the basic tracking, teaming, and focusing problems mentioned in the introduction. The end result is now the child can use more of his intellect. Rather than using so much effort and energy to perform the mechanical aspects of performing reading, he can now channel his energies into learning from reading.

At first this will occur only in short bursts and will be picked up by the Visagraph well before the same changes are revealed by testing that takes a longer than just a few minutes to complete. Only after six to 12 months using newly acquired skills and abilities may the gains that the child gets from having been involved in an optometric vision therapy program become consolidated or embedded enough that the child can use these new skills and abilities for long periods of time. Only then will the changes from the treatment reveal themselves on standardized testing.

1. The resultant hypothesis would rank the expected order of seeing changes in the tests, from earliest to latest, as followings: Gates Oral Reading Test – decoding only
2. Visagraph – difficulty change, no mechanics changes yet
3. Visagraph – mechanics changes at lower level demands
4. Visagraph – mechanics changes at higher level demands
5. Standardized reading test scores

Where Are We Now?

During the academic year of fall 2000 to spring 2001 we have begun working with a new group of fourth-graders. Some of the testing has been streamlined. Rather than working with randomly selected children from a pool of all children, the classroom teacher and the master fourth- grade teacher were asked to submit names of children they believed could benefit from the testing and treatment program. This single change has helped us gain significant support from the teachers and the administrators. From the pool of children identified with visual difficulties, children have been randomly chosen to participate in the treatment program. Those not chosen constitute the control group for those receiving treatment.

Standardized testing on the initial control and treatment groups will be done during the spring of 2001 and every spring for the next few years even though the children will have moved on to middle school. Results on these tests will be made available for analysis over the years. An attempt will be made to locate as many of the original groups as possible to repeat the Visagraph testing in the spring of 2001, 2002, 2003, and 2004.

Randomization Difficulties

When the randomization was done at the beginning of the study the group of children chosen to receive vision therapy were taken from the group of all children. The early screening showed that the prevalence of LRVPs was between 80% and 85%. Because the numbers were so high the samples were randomly taken from the entire student body. However, it is possible that some of the results did not show a great difference between the two groups because some of the children in the treatment group did not have primary vision problems. A post hoc analysis will be done to determine whether this might have been significant. Future designs should first cull from the general population of students those who have significant primary visual problems and then perform the randomization on that subgroup.

What Does the Future Hold?

The program will move in one of three directions. Plans are being made to expand initially to one additional school and then to expand over a 10-year period to all schools within the Baltimore City Public School system. Expansion would be dependent on the continued strengthening of the performance differences between the treatment and control groups. Launching a program from scratch at a second school with the benefit of our three years of experience at Harford Heights Elementary School should help to make the new program far more effective. If such a program is even more effective in another location then the evidence that vision therapy for LRVPs in inner-city school populations would be strengthened. At some point the evidence that the problem exists and that there is a safe and effective treatment for these problems may become overwhelming. Municipalities and school boards around the country and around the globe will need rational, cost-conscious plans and programs to address this major public health concern.

Where would funding for such a program come from? School-based optometric vision therapy may save significantly on the amount of money being spent on special education. Five to seven years from now we should be able to perform a retrospective study of the children in this study, comparing the treatment groups versus the control group to determine the level of special education services required by these children and calculate the actual costs to educate the different groups in our study. The Baltimore City Public Schools spend an average of $6800 per year on children who, under Public Law 94-142 and its regulations, require additional educational services over and above the base of $3100 per student per year for those not receiving extra services.

A detailed business plan of a program to bring this treatment to a major school district has been created, and projected gross cost per student served, including equipment, hiring, training, supervision, and all administrative costs, is between $1600 and $1750. This is a one-time expense per child with a learning-related visual problem. The $6800 is a recurring cost each year for as long as the child remains in school and needs extra educational and supportive services. In a case where a child is identified and treated in the fourth grade and if the optometric vision therapy reduces, on a conservative basis, by one-third the needs of the child served then the savings would be $13,586.40 per student served—more than an 8-to-1 return on investment. This assumes that on average these children stay in school only six years after this time. If either the treatment is more effective or the children on average stay in school longer, then the potential savings could be significantly higher.

References

1. Hoffman, Donald D., "Visual Intelligence – How We Create What We See", WW Norton and Company, 1998, ISBN 0-393-04669-9, p. 8 & p XII.

2. Lieberman, S., Cohen, A., "Validation Study of the New York State Optometric Association (NYSOA) Vision Screening Battery, American Journal of Optometry & Physiological Optics, vol. 62, No. 3. pp 165-168.

3. Cooper J., Duckman R., "Convergence insufficiency: incidence, diagnosis, and treatment." JAOA, 1978; 49:673-680.

4. Hoover D. The effects of using the ReadFast computer program on eye movement abilities as measured by the OBER2 Eye Movement Device. JOVD 28 Winter 1997, pp 227-234

5. Harris, Paul A, "The Prevalence of Visual Conditions in a Population of Juvenile Delinquents", OEPF 1989

6. Duane, A., "A new classification of the motor anomalies of the eye, based upon physiologic principles." Part 2. Pathology. Ann Ophthalmol 1897: 6:247-60.

7. Cooper J. Duckman R., "Convergence insufficiency incidence, diagnosis and treatment", J Am Optom Assoc 1978: 49:673-80.

8. Kent PR, Steeve JH, "Convergence insufficiency incidence among military personnel and relief by orthoptic methods." Mil Surg 1953; 114:202-5.

9. Norn MD., "Convergence insufficiency: incidence in ophthalmic practice results of orthoptic treatment." Acta Ophthalmol 1966; 44:132-8

10. Cohen, Lieberman, Stolzberg, Ritty, "The NYSOA Vision Screening Battery – A Total Approach", JAOA, November 1983, Vol. 7, pp 979-984.

11. Kulp, P.T., Schmidt, P., "Reliability of the NYSOA King-Devic Saccadic Eye Movement Test in Kindergartners and First Graders:, JAOA, September 1997, Vol. 68, No. 9, pp 589-595

12. Lieberman, Cohen, Rubin, "NYSOA K-D Test", JAOA, July 1983, Vol. 7, pp 631-637

13. Groffman, Sidney, "Visual Tracing", JAOA, Vol. 37, No. 2, February 1966, P. 139-141

14. Wold, Robert, "Screening Tests to be used by the Classroom Teacher", Academic Therapy Publications, 1970

15. Lowry, Raymond, "Handbook of Diagnostic Tests for the Developmental Optometrist", OEPF, 1970

16. Taylor, SE, Frackenpohl H, Pettee, JL, "Grade level norms for the components of the fundamental reading task." Research and Information Bulletin, No. 3, Huntington, NY: Educational Developmental Laboratories, Inc. 1960

17. Kraskin, Robert, "VT in Action", OEPF, 1965-1968.

18. Karni, Avi, "Adult Cortical Plasticity and Reorganization", Science & Medicine, January/February 1997.

19. Birnbaum, Martin, "Optometric Management of Nearpoint Vision Disorders", Butterworth-Heinemann, 1993, page 129

20. 20. Williams S, Simpson A, Silva PA., "Stereo acuity levels and vision problems from 7-11 years." Ophtahl Physiol Opt. Vol 8, 1988.

Acknowledgments

Assistance has been given by: Drs. Valerie Whittaker, Ted Sober, Ron Berger, Dana Taylor, Jason Sober, and Thelma Lombardi, Katherine McKearn, Emily Harris, Betty Francis, Cindy Hubbard, Carol Zimmerman, Sidney Chernick, Theresa Krejci, Dennis Hoover, Liz St. Ours, Jennifer Kungle, and Phyllis Lloyd. Essilor and Marchon/Marcolin as well as New City Optical have given additional assistance.

Statistics were done using SPSS version 10.0 for Windows. Because the variances for each test were made to be the same during the randomization process this fact was used in calculating the levels of significance. Means testing was done and compared for each of the treatment groups in each of the conditions against the controls. Analysis of variance testing yielded the quoted significance levels in each of the tables in this report.

Additional thanks to Molly Mullen who edited the first version of the paper and to Irwin Suchoff, Selwyn Super, and Lenny Press for their input.

Contact:
Paul Harris, OD, FCOVD, FACBO, FAAO, FNAP
Professor, Southern College of Optometry
1245 Madison Avenue
Memphis, TN 38104
Phone: 901-722-3273
E-mail: Paul.HarrisOD@gmail.com

Appendix A

Visual History

Name:_____ (M/F) Teacher:_____ Room:_____

Parent's Names:_____

Birth Date:_____ Has a grade been repeated (Y/N)?

Has glasses (Y/N)?

If yes, when are they worn (full time/school/home/close work/not worn)?

If no, did they ever have glasses? (Y/N)?

Besides screenings have you ever had a professional vision examination? (Y/N)?

    If yes, how long since your last exam? (<1 year / >1 and <2 years / >2 years)

Ask each of the following: Do you get or do you ever experience….

Headaches	Yes	No
Blurred distance sight	Yes	No
Blurred near sight	Yes	No
Double vision	Yes	No
Eyes feel tired	Yes	No
Eye hurt	Yes	No
Hold reading close	Yes	No
Hold reading far away	Yes	No
Close one eye	Yes	No
Cover one eye	Yes	No
Rub eyes excessively	Yes	No
Eyes red a lot of the time	Yes	No
Get lost when reading	Yes	No
Use your finger to keep your place	Yes	No
Bump into objects	Yes	No
Bothered by bright lights	Yes	No
Dislike reading	Yes	No

How much TV do you watch (<1 hour / 1> <3 hours / >3 hours)?

How well do you do in school (average / better than average / lower than average)?

Do you read (faster / slower / the same speed) as everyone else in your grade?

Do you understand (more / less / the same) as everyone else in your grade?

Appendix B

Baltimore Academy for Behavioral Optometry Learning-Related Visual Problems Curriculum (VT-II) for School-Based Vision Therapy

Session	Activity 1	Activity 2	Activity 3	Activity 4
1	Eye Control	Square Balance Board	Handball	Hart/Chart Near/Far Rock
2				
3		Walking Rail	Punch Ball	
4				
5			Thumb Ball	MAR
6	Chalk Board Circle Trace			
7			3 ways to catch	
8				
9	Chalk Board Racetracks			
10			Look and catch	
11	Chalkboard Double O's	Line Tracing		
12				
13			3 O's and catch	
14				
15			O's around head	
16	Comp. Video Saccades			
17			.	
18			Bunting	BAR
19	Coin Circles			
20				
21			"V" Bunting	
22		Mazes		
23			Half circles	
24	Visicare Disassociated Pointing			
25			Column Jumping	
26	Visicare Associated Pointing			
27				Keystone Fusion Games
28	Visicare Jump Ductions			

#				
29			Ann Arbor Letter Tracking	
30	Jumping			Near Vision Vectograms
31			Physiological Diplopia	
32	On table			
33				Vectogram Localization
34	Single – Stage 1		Brock String	
35				
36	Single – Stage 2		Bead Jumping	Vectogram Jump Ductions
37				
38	Slap Tap	Rotator Golf Tees	Bead Sliding	Vectogram BOP/BIM
39				
40			Bug on the string	Rotator O's
41		Rotator Tees with Ping Pong Balls		
42				
43		C-P Saccades	Bug on the wall	Comp Video Pursuits
44				
45				
46		Flashlight Pointing - 1 Light	ReadFast Comprehension Testing	Comp Vergence
47			Visualization – Arrow Jumping	
48	Cheiroscopic Tracing			Comp BI/BO JD
49			Visualization – Draw on Back	
50				Comp Directionality
51	Van Orden Stars	Flashlight Pointing 2 Lights		
52			Visualization – Mystery Bag	
53	Comp. Tachistoscope			Comp Visual/Motor Integration
54		Read Fast Moving Windows		
55			Visualization – Rotating Pictures	
56				Comp Auditory/ Visual Integration
57	Harry's Blocks			
58			Spelling Method	Comp Visual Scan
59				
60				Read Fast Tachistoscope